The Father's
Guide
to Birth, Babies, and Loud Children

SO-ADF-850

"Jim's life sounds like a daycare run amuck. I'm glad I'm not alone."
—**Anonymous from the Internet**

"Expectant dads are often told 'your life is about to completely change!' Which is useful to know, but not terribly specific... many wonder what, exactly, that might mean. Hoehn's laugh-out-loud explanations provide enlightening details about the many different ways in which dad's life will become sleepless, loud, frenetic, messy, and yes, more wonderful, with the arrival of children."
—**Lisa Falk, Senior Librarian, Los Angeles Public Library**

"(Jim Hoehn's book) offers a practical, often humorous look at how fathers can survive the early childhood years with at least some amounts of sanity."
—**Leader-Telegram (Eau Claire, Wisconsin)**

"I haven't laughed this hard at family life since 'Everybody Loves Raymond' went into summer repeats. Jim's tales of parenting come from his heart and strike our funny bone. It's a laugh a sentence."
—**Gina Hernandez, Madison, Wis.**

"Jim Hoehn has nailed it! This is the funniest and most clever book on being a dad I've ever read. Best of all, every word of it rings true. You won't want to put this book down."
—**Carson Cooper, Radio Margaritaville**

"Jim Hoehn hit a home run with this hilarious look at how fathers can attempt to survive the scary-yet-rewarding journey through parenthood. From treating pregnant wives with the proper degree of reverence to solving the baby dress code riddle to dealing with the every-day stress of raising children without losing your cool, this book offers a refreshing, comedy filled look at what to expect of – and how to enjoy – becoming a dad."
—**Julian Emerson, Eau Claire, Wis.**

"If Spock is the doctor of parenting, then Hoehn really should be his physician assistant. His tales and insights on being a father bring a little levity and a lot of laughter to the process."
—**Fred Benz, Madison, Wis.**

"A must-read for all of the edgy mothers and fathers who feel one public outburst from their wee one tarnishes the parenting process forever. After reading this book, who are they kidding? Hoehn shows us that childish behavior is the stuff memories are made of."
—**Lisa Brudos, Madison, Wis.**

"The Father's Guide made my wife laugh uncontrollably. What's Jim's secret?"
—**Rob Hernandez, Madison, Wis.**

"I think the book is hilarious. Around our house we have only two children, but often find ourselves laughing to keep from crying. I was glad to laugh (hysterically, I might add) at someone else's circus for a while! It's comforting to know there's someone else out there shameless enough to share silly stories. We were both glad to see we're not the only ones! What a comic relief!"
—**Amanda Carter**

los angeles, california
www.pgpress.com

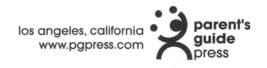

parent's guide press

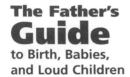

The Father's
Guide
to Birth, Babies,
and Loud Children

7   12   29   34   45   AA

Edwin E. Steussy, CEO and Publisher
Lars W. Peterson, Project Editor
Michael P. Duggan, Graphic Artist/
Cartoonist

PO Box 461730
Los Angeles CA 90046

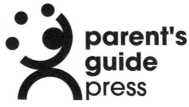

parent's
guide
press

The Father's Guide
to Birth, Babies, and Loud Children

Contents

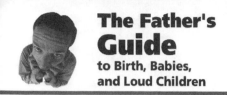

The Father's
Guide
to Birth, Babies,
and Loud Children

Contents

Contents

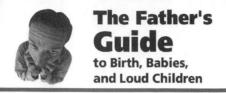

The Father's
Guide
to Birth, Babies,
and Loud Children

Acknowledgements

This book is dedicated to my wife and best friend, Karen Gray-Hoehn, whose love and tireless effort put a stable foundation under the asylum. It also is dedicated to Hayley, Tyler and Colin, the daily embodiment of joie de vivre.

Thanks to Kathy Mangold, Edie Boatman and Todd Kotlarek at MetroPARENT for the opportunity to mix my metaphors and misplace my modifiers in the interest of family journalism, which is cheaper than therapy.

Thanks to the staff at the Pavlic Women's Center at Elmbrook Memorial Hospital, Brookfield, Wisconsin, for their help with a remedial student.

The Father's
Guide
to Birth, Babies,
and Loud Children

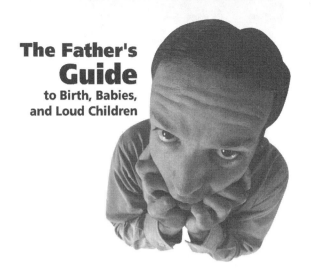

Introduction

The reason this book is called "A Father's Guide to Birth, Babies, and Loud Children" supposedly is based on my wealth of accumulated parental knowledge thanks to having three children within a 5-year-span, now between the ages of 3 and 7.

If that was truly the case, this book would be titled "Pull My Finger," the extent of my fatherly knowledge, lovingly passed from one generation to the next by well-intentioned males.

At least that was the depth of my knowledge going into our first pregnancy.

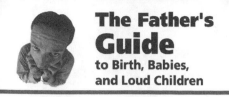

Introduction

Now, as a battle-tested veteran of the diaper wars, I have learned enough about daily parenting to realize I probably know less than when I started.

From the parental perspective, not a single day goes by without some sort of new challenge.

Everyday elements taken for granted, such as sleep, organization and punctuality will become things of the past, buried like the Day Care Center of Pompeii under layers and layers of changing priorities.

Your house will be under constant siege by the legions of germs that swirl throughout the world of kiddom. Coughs, colds, sneezes and sniffles will be your constant companions.

You will be confronted with skin rashes the likes of which, according to home reference books, were last seen on the decks of Columbus' sailing ships.

Reading material will consist largely of medicine dosage charts and child-safety recall notices. You will hear the phrase "not covered by insurance" more often than a good song on the radio.

Disarray will officially become your style of interior decor. You will learn to speak fluent laundry and master the art of stain camouflage.

The broken wheel on a 59-cent plastic car will trigger hours of sobbing, chest-heaving hysteria while stitches and X-rays will be heroically faced with silent stoicism.

A penny saved will invariably turn out to be a penny eaten. If tears were nickels, you could bail out the Enron Corp.

Raising children is not a learning curve, it is a roller coaster of the gut-busting, scream-inducing variety with dizzying highs, terrifying lows and stomach-churning drops and climbs interspersed at every opportunity with head-snapping turns.

And, even though you are theoretically safe and secure in your own little cart, you definitely are not in control as life whizzes past you in the proverbial blur. Sometimes the best you can do is hang on and enjoy the ride.

But, when you have come to a stop and used those few fleeting seconds to regain your breath and your senses, there is something that makes you want to climb back aboard and do it again and again and again.

Introduction

What becomes more and more apparent as each day of never-ending disasters unfolds is the painfully obvious difference between the male take on parenting versus that of the female viewpoint.

Although the theory of gender difference could easily be substantiated by the head count at a *Three Stooges* film festival, a recent spate of tax-funded scientific studies by a bunch of lab coat-wearing academia nuts who wouldn't know a Curley from a Shemp has validated the findings.

From the initial discovery of pregnancy, men and women react differently for one very good reason – women do all the work. Their bodies change, their hormones rage, and their moods swing like a New Year's Eve dance band.

The role of a guy during pregnancy is basically one of support, a sort of maternity caddie who, if smart, keeps his mouth shut, carries the heavy bag and selects the proper club when asked.

But the pregnancy period is not so much fatherhood as perhaps spousal-hood or maybe partner-hood. After the birth of the baby, however, this is where fatherhood revs its testosterone-based engine and shifts into high gear as you move from spectator to participant.

Don't get me wrong. Parenting is without a doubt hard work and at times overwhelming, but the benefits are beyond compare. Kids are a source of continual amazement and enjoyment, as well as the key to the long-locked toy chest of immaturity.

All the childhood favorites that made being a kid the world's greatest job description, but were eventually tucked away under the constraints of adult acceptability, are once again fair game.

Fireworks, monster trucks, tree climbing, hand-in-the-armpit noises, ball games and, yes, finger pulling, can be trotted out under the guise of parental involvement.

With a little luck, these tricks of the testosterone trade can be used to subtly augment such concepts as honesty, integrity and fairness, sort of like using the Man From Nantucket as an introduction to the Man From La Mancha.

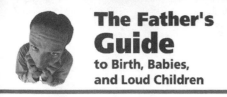

Introduction

About This Book

That is also why this book is written the way it is.

It is for those of us whose daily flight through parenthood is by the seat of our Levis as opposed to some well-organized, theory-backed knowledge of creating perfect children.

Those are the people to whom I turned in my quest for accurate and informative detail. Dozens of friends, co-workers and mildly interested strangers – both male and female – stepped forward with their own tales of pregnancy and parenting, offering embarrassing family tales of bodily fluids and functions with total disregard for discretion or spousal wrath.

The simple truth is I know more people like that and families like ours than I do officially sanctioned childhood researchers.

Based on titles alone, many people who put pen to paper in the interest of perfect parenting apparently have never actually had children or they are simply delusional.

Royalty checks aside, I'm sure many of these books are well-intentioned. Some may even be read.

I know in our own house with the aforementioned three kids under the age of 8, approximately 7.2 tons of unfolded laundry and a daily schedule of being behind schedule, there is nothing like taking an entire afternoon to leisurely wade through a 200-page book that basically tells you that your life, and your house, is a mess.

Noticeably absent from the bookstore offerings on how to be the perfect parent were reality-based publications on the day-to-day battle with life itself.

Not one single, solitary book dealt with "How To Make Laundry Disappear When The Doorbell Rings." No author touched on, "The Inconspicuous Removal of Snot In Public." No brave literary soul ventured down the path of "Dorkiness, A Hereditary Problem."

Hopefully, this book will help fill that untouched void or, if not, at least prop up the end table with the broken leg.

Parental time constraints also are one of the primary reasons why many of the following chapters are relatively short. Our lifestyle leaves no more time to write than you have to read. It is a book that not only will not be embarrassed to be left on the bathroom counter, it would consider it a place of honor, especially if it shares the space with a week's worth of sports sections. If your copy eventually has a coffee ring stain on the cover, so much the better.

Any and all advice, information or disinformation contained herein is based primarily on my own experience, which revolves around the trial-and-error method of parenting, with the emphasis on error.

From our first trip home from the maternity ward, I have, for better or worse, tried to take an active, roll-up-your-sleeves approach of on the job training as opposed to relying on abstract theory and TV talk-show psychobabble.

As with my monthly magazine columns, much of this book is based on our three children – Hayley, Tyler and Colin. I know, I know. Great. An entire book based on, yawn, other people's kids. But it's not so much about them, but what they represent – the pressure and pleasures involved with childhood with which the average beleaguered parent can identify. To me, Hayley, Tyler and Colin are simply the voices and actions of kids everywhere whose main job is to make nitwits like me into semi-reliable, if somewhat embarrassing, parents.

In addition to their daily role in exposing my lack of parental acumen, our children were instrumental in the slow and unsteady progress of this book, taking an active role in the daily editorial grind.

One telephone conversation with the editor was overheard by Hayley, whose lofty standing as a first grade reader-in-training obviously qualified her to offer literary advice.

As soon as I hung up the phone, she began the question and answer session.

Hayley: "Are you an author?"

Dad: "Nope, just a writer."

Hayley: "So, you're not famous or anything."

Dad: "Nope, I just write stuff now and then."

Hayley: "What's this book stuff?"

Dad: "Oh, nothing. Just talking with someone."

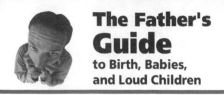

The Father's Guide
to Birth, Babies,
and Loud Children

Introduction

Hayley: "Who's going to illustrate it?"

Dad: "I don't know. Would it be better with pictures?"

Hayley: "Yes. Would there be a picture on the cover?"

Dad: "Probably"

Hayley: "Is it a funny book?"

Dad: "Maybe. I hope so."

Hayley: "Then the cover should have a picture of you like in the morning. You know, in your underwear with your hair sticking up. That's pretty funny."

From the standpoint of cover art, consider yourself fortunate. In terms of editorial content and practical advice, somebody has to extend the literary finger to be pulled.

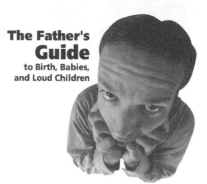

The Father's Guide
to Birth, Babies,
and Loud Children

Chapter One
Ready, Set, Go!

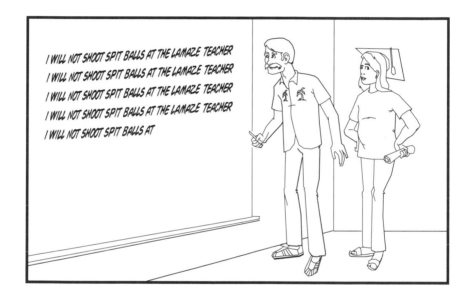

I WILL NOT SHOOT SPIT BALLS AT THE LAMAZE TEACHER
I WILL NOT SHOOT SPIT BALLS AT THE LAMAZE TEACHER
I WILL NOT SHOOT SPIT BALLS AT THE LAMAZE TEACHER
I WILL NOT SHOOT SPIT BALLS AT THE LAMAZE TEACHER
I WILL NOT SHOOT SPIT BALLS AT

We're Pregnant

As a concession to chronological correctness, as well as an admission that a sportswriting career is not exactly the equivalent of a medical degree in terms of maternity-related knowledge, I referred to an invaluable, not to mention free, source of information on pregnancy while writing this book; our own dog-eared, hospital-provided, three-ring binder, "Pregnancy, Childbirth, Parenting."

Ironically, the information provided by our hospital begins with the section, "Becoming Pregnant." I'm guessing that if you're holding your own copy of an official three-ring notebook, or something similar, you've already got that part figured out.

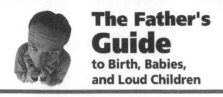
Chapter One

Still, it's nice a gesture on the part of the hospital folks just in case a lifelong exposure to street corners, locker rooms, dormitories, barracks and Naugahyde-covered backseats was not sufficient to provide the basic information.

Although the inclusively correct phrase is, "We're pregnant," men, no matter how interested or excited, will never be more than the second to know. The actual discovery of "I'm pregnant" is solely the domain of the expectant mother. At some point, however, the information usually is communicated by the female half of the twosome that tangoed.

To avoid one of those unnecessary speed bumps in the road of marital bliss, it is best this information be conveyed in the most straightforward manner possible with little or no room for misinterpretation.

For example, phrasing this life-changing information with a somewhat ambiguous, "I have something important to tell you," can have different meanings dependent upon gender. When presented from female to male, this statement invariably conjures up images of a wrecked car or the possibility that she is running off to the Caribbean with a graduate student turned lawn care expert.

If the subject is simply stated, "We're expecting," the response 9 times out of 10 will be, "Expecting what?" triggering a marital spat worthy of Judge Judy's involvement.

In most instances, the news should be delivered with a simple, straightforward, "I'm pregnant," preferably when the intended recipient does not have a mouthful of anything on which he can choke.

Regardless of how the news is delivered, the stunning announcement is the basis behind the phrase, "pregnant pause," a woefully inadequate description of the initial reaction to pregnancy in which all the air seems to be sucked out of the room.

In my case, I was seated on the edge of our bed when Karen told me she was pregnant with our first child. An hour later, I was still seated on the edge of the bed, mouth open, eyes glazed over with every synapse misfiring as I tried to process the information.

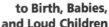

Ready, Set, Go!

Wildly vacillating responses such as shock, panic and dizziness came later, accompanied by thoughts of skyrocketing college tuition, the likelihood of never owning a two-seat convertible and the possibility of a one-way ticket to Paraguay.

Eventually, I settled into kind of a consistent state of excitement. Although definitely unsure about the changes in our life that I knew were coming, I was eagerly awaiting the due date. Then again, I wasn't the one throwing up every morning.

Pregnancy-related news is hard to contain and different people obviously have different approaches as to when, what and to whom the information is provided.

Some expectant parents immediately begin to beat the jungle drums of pregnancy, sending the message as far and wide as possible. From day one, every thought, action and conversation is dedicated toward the pregnancy and the arrival of the baby.

For those who favor an early and active approach, any male-dominated room, such as a den, home office or TV-watching hideaway is quickly converted into a nursery, nine months ahead of the due date, but never too soon in terms of color coordinated, Pooh-themed walls, curtains and bedspreads. Proudly displayed softball trophies are relegated to a cardboard box in the garage rafters.

Infant clothes are organized, folded and hung in dressers and closets in anticipation of that all-important first week's wardrobe.

Baby dishes, including rubber-tipped spoons and sippy cups, move to the front of their respective cupboards. An army of sterilized baby bottles and nipples is mobilized to greet the newcomer.

Others opt for the more restrained, low-key style, subscribing to the theory that you don't talk about a no-hitter in progress. In that case, pregnancy plans are carried out in relative secrecy, if they are carried out at all. In our case, we delayed the feeling of panic for as long as possible, holding off on most of the home organizing until after the baby arrived. Some seven years later, we still haven't caught up.

When it comes to offending friends and relatives, delivering pregnancy news is a matter of personal choice, rather than a matter of right or wrong, which you will invariably be.

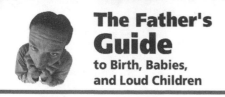

Chapter One

A Little Knowledge Is A Dangerous Thing

First-time expectant parents all have one thing in common. When it comes to childbirth, they know absolutely nothing.

Zero, zip, zilch, nada.

Of course, it's not your fault that until now your only knowledge of delivery has to do with dinner. Pizzas you've had, kids you haven't.

But there is nothing you can do about it. The only experience that counts in this case is experience you don't have.

That's not to say you're on your own, however. Family, friends and neighborhood busybodies are quick to offer a steady stream of well-intentioned, if totally confusing, advice.

For every delivery room fairy tale ("she was in and out in seven minutes, knitted two booties and sang 'South Pacific' with the doctor") another well-informed family member is quick to leap in with the story ("I know it's true, I saw it on Geraldo") of some woman who was in labor for 37 days and ate only ice chips before giving birth to identical twins 10 days apart.

Of course, these are the female versions of delivery room stories and are more of the what-you-can-expect nature.

Men's versions usually are more after-the-fact and not as medically detailed ("I tell you, it was nip and tuck there for a minute. I thought for sure I was going to miss my tee time.").

Without firsthand experience, however, it's almost impossible to tell good advice from bad. But then again, it doesn't matter. None of it will apply to your specific situation.

In our case, a little classroom learning proved to be the best option. That's how we ended up with the three-ring binder from the hospital.

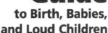

Class Is In Session

One of the most informative sources when dealing from a position of blissful baby ignorance is the ever-popular prenatal class, where expectant mothers take detailed notes and expectant fathers discretely glance at their watches to see if they can at least catch the last quarter of Monday Night Football.

Our hospital, like many others, offered a variety of classes dealing with almost every facet of pregnancy. From a male standpoint, if much of your college time was spent at fraternity parties and happy hours instead of medical school, prenatal classes are the real-life version of the book, *Pregnancy for Dummies.*

Much like a college course of study, our curriculum centered around a core group of a four-class series collectively known as "Childbirth Preparation."

It was recommended that these classes begin during the seventh month of pregnancy in order to undo the seven months of totally irrelevant misinformation provided by every other person with whom you have come in contact up to that point.

Most of the class attendees were couples, bound together not only by pregnancy, but the fear of the unknown. As such, the instructor's first task was simply to put the class at ease and try not to laugh out loud when bombarded with the idiotic questions of the truly panic-stricken.

The instructor of one of the first classes referred to the initial two-hour session as the "sensory overload tour," where expectant parents are inundated with pregnancy-related information, a basic primer in what to do and what not to do. Or, as she put it, "this is where the fun begins."

It's also where I write little short snippets about some of the pregnancy class highlights, sort of a Cliff Notes approach. If you want more detailed information, I'm sure there's probably an opening in a classroom near you.

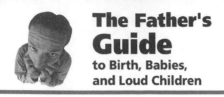
Chapter One

First Things First

One of the first discussion sessions in our class dealt with some of the changes associated with pregnancy. Subjects brought up by male class members as changes they had noticed in their partner included tiredness, more frequent need for a rest room, mood swings, swelling and outright fear.

Expectant mothers mentioned an overall feeling of anxiety, leg cramps, trouble sleeping, back aches, skin problems, clumsiness, morning sickness, heartburn, constipation, trouble putting on shoes, forgetfulness, food cravings and the need for nesting.

Other than those few minor inconveniences, which apparently vary from occasionally to all day, every day, most of the maternity situation is a relatively smooth sail.

In addition to being informative, the group setting allowed for easy conversational voicing of concerns, at the same time reassuring each couple that they were not the only ones whose stress level was higher than Bill Gates' credit card limit.

As each troubling topic was mentioned, it was greeted with nodding heads and knowing smiles of familiarity. It was not so much that misery loved company, it just needed affirmation.

During a discussion on tiredness, one guy risked being put on conversational probation for the rest of his life when he complained that "he was the tired one because she gets up all the time to go the bathroom and she wakes me up every time she flushes the toilet."

If the proverbial looks could, indeed, kill, he would have been instantly ventilated by the angry glare of every woman in the room.

The episode did emphasize, however, one of the cardinal rules of male self-preservation: Never, ever try to out-complain a pregnant woman.

Fatigue

Regarding tiredness, the instructor, who herself was a mother as well as a recent grandmother, encouragingly told the class that pregnancy was the first step on the "slippery slope of sleep deprivation and that it is going to last for a very, very, very long time."

Even in the initial classroom sessions, the fatigue was physically noticeable. It was like sitting in a room full of raccoons. Based on the dark circles under the eyes of everyone in the class, everyone was becoming well acquainted with pregnancy-related insomnia.

As with most discomforts associated with pregnancy, expectant mothers bear the brunt of the sleeplessness. While she is struggling to properly place the 27 pillows needed for comfort and readying for another night of several dozen trips to the bathroom, you can always opt for a quiet night on the couch

The difficulties of getting a good night's rest during pregnancy pale in comparison to the sleepless nights after the baby arrives. No one in our house has slept since 1994.

The Nearest Restroom, Quick

Frequent urination was another widely acknowledged topic and one with which we had a great deal of first-hand experience.

When my wife was pregnant for the first time, we combined business and pleasure on a trip to New York City, where I had previously lived and worked for a couple years. As such, I was able to personally and efficiently conduct much of the sightseeing tour, which was interrupted either every block or every 13 minutes by the need to find an available restroom.

One of the main problems with a walking tour of Manhattan is that you could not nonchalantly wander off Broadway and in to a fast-food restaurant or other plumbing-equipped establishment and simply use the bathroom. In each and every instance, use of a restroom required a purchase of some sort.

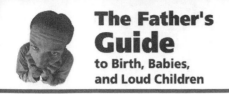
Chapter One

As a result, in a four-day span I bought, and drank, roughly 319 small sodas. Thankfully, I could wait until we returned to the hotel.

Over the course of the pregnancy, you will know where every bathroom is in every shopping mall for miles around, which gas stations require an outdoor key, and family trips will be planned around the rest area icons on state highway maps.

Remembering the exact location and amenities of every bathroom in the hemisphere apparently occupies the bulk of the memory bank as almost everything else is forgotten.

Memory, What Memory?

To the non-pregnant, the sudden advent of forgetfulness is a hard-to-explain pregnancy phenomenon. Intelligent, successful women whose entire life is based on organization suddenly become a one-person scavenger hunt constantly on the prowl for misplaced items.

A good friend of mine, whose business success belies our jointly shared college rugby days, referred to this condition as "pregnancy Alzheimer's." His wife was an accountant whose daily approach to everything was based on organization and attention to detail. When she was pregnant, however, it appeared, he implied, as if she had been the one who had endured one too many rugby collisions.

Which brings up another simple rule of survivability. Do not, in mixed company, ever refer to your pregnant wife as "the mayor of Airhead City," especially when she still handles the family checkbook.

Menu Changes

One of the first items subjected to pregnancy-related memory loss is the list of culinary likes and dislikes.

There is absolutely no rhyme or reason to some of the food cravings associated with pregnancy. Lifelong favorite foods suddenly become unpalatable while others, previously placed in the daily food group known as "gross," become a daily requirement.

Another friend, whose wife was pregnant with their first child while I was writing this book, was happy to serve as a culinary consultant. To put some of his wife's pre-pregnancy food choices in perspective, she is 1) from California; 2) an artist; and 3) a vegetarian. During her pregnancy, however, she suddenly developed an insatiable craving for bacon. To maintain her Left Coast artistic aura she pointed out that it was not *she* who craved the bacon, but the baby, whose wishes she, of course, had to abide by.

But, as somewhat of a politically correct concession, she only ate the meaty parts of the bacon. Her husband, in an act of thoughtfulness, would carefully and painstakingly hack away the fatty parts to present his pseudo-vegetarian wife a finely trimmed sliver of meaty bacon. Because he originally hailed from the Midwest, the leftover parts did not go to waste.

Of course, there always is the chance that the platter of bacon, as well as anything else that might be carried or balanced, could suddenly drop like a wind-blown Wallenda, winding up in a puddle on the non stain proof carpeting left over from the pre-childhood era.

Lack Of Coordinated Effort

The sudden loss of muscle control and balance by expectant mothers is simply known by the non-medical school term of pregnancy-related clumsiness, which strikes different people at different times and in different forms.

During one pregnancy, Karen cleaned out an entire set of drinking glasses, one dropped glass at a time. And, it was not like she was trying to subtly dispose of a set of my old college happy hour mugs. She actually was quite fond of this particular set.

My sister-in-law didn't have the dropsies so much as the stumbles. When she was pregnant, she tumbled down more flights of stairs than an entire troupe of Chinese gymnasts. And, in case you have never noticed, the body construction of an expectant mother does not usually lend itself to cartwheels.

In addition to clumsiness, physical changes in the body also lead to movement restriction, which is not always a bad thing.

When Karen was pregnant with our daughter, Hayley, our first child, we used to sneak off for an occasional 9-hole round of golf for both the sake of exercise and a breath of fresh air.

The farther along she got in her pregnancy, the better she golfed. As her stomach got larger and heavier, she was forced to take a very, very compact back swing and also was forced to keep her head down on each shot.

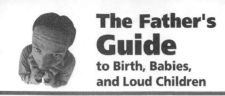

Chapter One

The result was a dramatic, short-but-accurate improvement in her golf game.

If your main goal is to simply shave a couple strokes off your game, I would, however, as a matter of practicality, recommend golf lessons rather than becoming pregnant. Then again, if you have three or four children in close succession, your wife might be breaking par on a regular basis.

After touching on as many other pregnancy-related topics as one two-hour session would allow, the first class ended with a group demonstration of quickness and dexterity as the entire female delegation briskly waddled en masse for the nearest restroom.

Part of the second class in the series dealt with such things as pain management and medication, including the passing along of an old maternity ward joke.

Q: "When is the best time to get an epidural?

A: "When you find out you're pregnant.

The women in the class seemed to find this infinitely more hilarious than did the men.

Other parts of the curriculum included lifestyle changes, growth and development of the baby, dietary requirements and pregnancy fitness and exercise.

Diet

As with any voice of health-related authority, our instructor echoed the written mantra of the three-ring binder and urged expectant mothers to "Eat Healthy!"

Basically that means eating like you know you're supposed to, but rarely do. Our hospital divided dietary requirements into six food groups: the bread, cereal, rice or pasta group; vegetable group; fruit group; milk, yogurt, cheese group; meat, poultry, fish, dry beans, eggs or nuts group; and, finally, the fats, oils and sweets group.

Each good-for-you category had suggested serving sizes and numbers. As expected, the fats, oils and sweets group, which included butter, soft drinks, candy and sweet desserts, simply said, "Use sparingly."

As a result, many expectant fathers quickly learn the art of junk food subterfuge, eating properly and 'supportingly' at home, but after leaving the house alone, immediately stopping at the nearest Quickee Mart for a sugar fix. If that is the case, make sure you get rid of the evidence. Many a marital spat has ensued upon the discovery of an automotive back seat full of Snickers wrappers, doughnut boxes and fully-sugared soda cans.

Pregnant women also are urged to refrain from drinking alcoholic beverages. For many women, abstinence from alcohol is not nearly as frustrating or limiting as yet another pregnancy-related restriction. It is probably not a good idea to keep reminding her how convenient it is to have a designated driver in the house for the next nine months.

Exercise

Expectant fathers also get the long end of the stick in the pregnancy-related exercise department. Our hospital binder contained several pages of exercises that pregnant women were urged to do on a regular basis. Nowhere did it mention that expectant fathers were required to do even one additional sit-up, much less a round of pelvic tilts.

In addition to the basic level of hospital-provided information, many health-care facilities or libraries have additional books, tapes or classes on exercise during pregnancy. These make great gifts and can be charged at the same time you buy yourself the $79 coffee table book on the world's greatest golf holes. Even though you don't have to do the exercises, it's the thought that counts.

Diapering

As simple as it may seem, one half of an entire class dealt with diapering techniques. Participants were asked to bring a doll of some sort on which to practice. As many first-time parents do not have a stash of dolls laying around, practice diapers have been applied to everything from Kermit the Frog to Power Rangers to Teddy Bears.

Once the baby is born, you'll quickly get a handle on diaper changing for one simple reason: you have no choice.

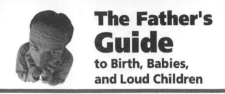
Chapter One

Along with diaper changing was a swaddling demonstration. Swaddling basically is the technique of securely wrapping a baby in a blanket, which has an immediate calming and comforting effect. After a few rounds of swaddling practice, you realize that with the required folding and tucking, the procedure is remarkably similar to that used in making a burrito. The goal in both instances is to keep the contents inside.

Car Seats

Proper use of car seats also was covered because at some point you have to bring the baby home. Many states require car seats for infants and children, which means you and the baby can't leave the hospital without one.

Infant car seats come in a wide range of styles based on height, weight and age and it is critical to select the correct model for your child. After that, the operational aspects of a particular car seat with its twisted straps, buckles and snaps can be easily mastered with three or four years of daily practice. Just as you have the infant car seat down pat, it's time to move to a booster chair.

The Two-Minute Tour

A tour of the hospital also was part of the classroom instruction. Expectant parents visited the maternity ward and viewed what our hospital referred to as "birth suites." Although the introduction helps, touring the birth suite as part of a classroom group differs greatly from when you're there for the real deal.

The difference between the tour and the maternity visit is like trying to compare a leisurely walk across an empty football practice field to being thrown into the lineup in the middle of an NFL game. Either way, at least you know where the stadium is.

Open Door Policy

One final sage bit of advice, which seems like common sense and somewhat trivial, was offered by the instructor based on her first-hand experience with frantic expectant parents.

Ready, Set, Go!

Be sure you know which door to use when you arrive at the hospital for the big event. A large hospital has dozens of entrances and exits, many of which are locked after certain hours or which are used for other purposes, such as doctors rushing out to their mid-afternoon tee times.

When the due date finally comes due, you do not want to be circling the parking lot like a last-minute holiday mall shopper while the expectant mother finally is fulfilling her expectations.

Other Classes

Other classes offered by our hospital included a refresher course for those parents who've had somewhat of a gap between children, a sibling preparation course for parents and children, breastfeeding and the active mom, childbirth express, infant CPR and infant massage.

Many hospitals offer a similar range of classes with varying and accommodating schedules. Some hospitals or healthcare facilities cram the entire curriculum into one marathon weekend session. Rest assured that when this one-time approach is selected, the weekend chosen will turn out to be 80 degrees and sunny.

A general rule of thumb is that help and information is available on almost any topic in a format that can be comfortably tailored to individual needs, situations and beliefs.

Pregnancy advice is like any other topic where you personally have limited background or skill. If your sink clogs up and the foul-smelling goop you pour down the drain doesn't meet advertised expectations, you call a plumber. If, after three dropped wrenches, four skinned knuckles and roughly 700 swear words, you still have not identified the source of the ka-thunk sound in the engine compartment, common sense eventually overrides stubbornness and sends you in the direction of a certified auto mechanic. In other words, offset what you don't know by turning to those who do.

Above all, if there is a problem or concern of any kind, call your doctor. Don't hesitate. Don't put it off. Don't be embarrassed about asking what you think is a stupid question. It probably is, but they've heard them all. Mostly from us.

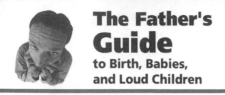
Chapter One

Finances

Many pre-natal classes provide a session on finances and expenses related to pregnancy, infancy and toddlers, continuing right on up through teenagers who want candy-apple red convertibles. Purchasing the first pack of disposable diapers hammers home the point that raising children is not without cost.

Because most of my financial expertise revolved around the nickel-dime betting strength of a three-Jack poker hand, this was welcome advice. With a few simple monthly checkbook adjustments, each of our kids now has a realistic shot of eventually attending the tech school of their choice.

A sports writing colleague, also wrestling with the daily costs of child raising, offered perhaps the best bit of advice on how to secure your financial future – write a parenting book that sells for $1 that no family in mainland China can live without and you are instantly a billionaire.

What he really means is, turn to someone other than a sportswriter for family financial advice. Lottery tickets are not your best option.

Woe Is Us: Expectant Fathers

In addition to subjects and situations more readily identifiable with and by expectant mothers, some discussion also was devoted to a topic called expectant fathers' syndrome, which sounds like an eligibility requirement for some sort of down-on-your-luck government disability plan.

According to our official pregnancy binder, which devoted a total of one entire paragraph to the role of expectant fathers, hanging out with other guys is a recommended part of the pregnancy experience.

Included in the in-depth paragraph of instruction was the following bit of sage advice. "As a father, it is important to get support from other men as well. Your father, brothers and male friends are all resources for support during good and bad times. Draw on them regularly."

Ready, Set, Go!

As such, feel free to schedule such things as golf outings, poker games and bachelor parties to help you deal with the pressure of pregnancy. After all, you're only following doctor's orders.

Another portion of the four-class series dealt with the hands-on role of the expectant father. This is where you got down to the nitty-gritty of practical application, sort of the shop class of pregnancy, learning about the actual labor process, including breathing techniques and your so-called role as pregnancy coach.

Even if you've paid attention in class, when the time comes, several months' worth of prenatal information will immediately dissolve into an unusable blur when faced with the sterilized pressure of a hospital delivery room. Such things as simple breathing techniques immediately are erased from memory at the mere suggestion of actual labor.

When Hayley was born, my own misguided effort went something like, "Exhale, inhale, count to seven (or is it three?), push, relax, count. No wait, start again. Take a deep breath. Not that deep."

Had I been teaching Karen to play the bagpipes, these instructions would have been extremely useful. As bedside childbirth assistance, however, this was not the well-rehearsed rhythm we had practiced in class.

If I was, indeed, the pregnancy coach, our team was not going to the Delivery Room Super Bowl.

Looking back, however, I think this is the precise reason why men are encouraged to take part in prenatal classes. From a learning standpoint, you will retain no more than you did from college physics, but trying to remember what you can't remember will keep you occupied while mother and doctor team up for the actual delivery.

The best you can hope for is to stay out of the way and not trip over any electrical cords.

We have now been through the delivery of three wonderful, healthy babies and I'm still not sure how we did it, although I'm sure Karen has a much better idea than I do.

It has something to do with doing all the work.

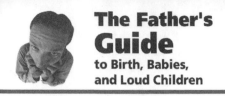
Chapter One

Good Things Come In Threes

For ease in record keeping, pregnancy is divided into three segments, cleverly, if simplistically, named The First Trimester; The Second Trimester and The Third Trimester.

As the numerical progression indicates, the successive trimesters span the entire pregnancy with the first trimester being the early stages, logically followed by the second and third trimesters.

Based on that premise, the whole thing is as easy as 1-2-3, for those of you scoring at home.

Each trimester has associated with it various changes in the expectant mother as well as developmental stages of the baby.

Because the changes are affecting the mother and baby, the role of the expectant father in this part of the pregnancy is that of an observer. And, if smart, a silent one.

Much of the medical description, including fertilization, female body parts and fetal development was, when you think about it, covered in eighth-grade health class. If you had paid attention instead of shooting spitwads through a hollowed-out Bic pen, you would recall such terminology as uterus, placenta and amniotic fluid and wouldn't need prenatal instruction.

As a concession to all academic backgrounds, our hospital binder provided an easy-to-read and easy-to-follow guide to each of the three trimesters.

Despite going through three pregnancies and being in the delivery room for each of our three children, I could not exactly pass a test on fetal development. In fact, I couldn't even bluff my way through a freshman term paper on the subject, much less come up with a semi-usable, fact-based book chapter, so I won't try.

The reason for much of the unfamiliarity is basically a case of out of sight, out of mind as the baby obviously is developing inside the mother. You cannot see the developmental changes as they take place, although the mother can feel various aspects of growth and development.

You're sort of out of the loop on this one for a while. Just think of it as the first time your child will do something of consequence when you're not watching. It is a skill they will continue to develop until finally reaching expert status as teenagers.

Ready, Set, Go!

There are many different types of books, magazine articles and web sites dealing with fetal development ranging from basic guidelines to detailed medical explanations. Our hospital binder covered 99 percent of anything you need to know in six concise pages, complete with line drawings. It was the perfect study guide for a male attention span honed on several decades of comic book reading.

There also are a variety of tests and procedures performed during each of the trimesters, including such things as determining blood type and screening for various diseases. Most hospitals have a straight-forward timetable for required tests and all you have to do is follow the schedule.

It is easier than trying to remember when to change the oil and rotate the tires on your car.

Picture This

One of the few procedures in which the expectant father can share also is one of the most fascinating and, for many, the most emotional. That procedure is the ultrasound, which basically shows a picture of the fetus.

During the ultrasound a scanning device is placed on the abdomen of the expectant mother to create the image of the baby, which is shown on a monitor or TV screen.

In our case, Karen laid down on a table and the doctor and nurse squirted some sort of brown goop onto her stomach. The doctor then slowly ran a gizmo that looked a lot like a computer mouse back and forth over her stomach.

The black-and-white images were then shown on the monitor where both Karen and I could watch. And, if there's one thing most men can do, it's watch a TV screen.

The unfolding images bore a strong resemblance to one of those ship-wreck-hunting shows on the Discovery Channel, where a camera-equipped, robot-controlled submersible trolls the ocean floor while beaming its barely discernible images to the screen on the mother ship above.

As the doctor navigated his way across Karen's stomach, I half expected to see the remains of the *Titanic*, or at least the frozen face of Leonardo DiCaprio, appear on the monitor before us. Suddenly, the picture on the screen evolved from an empty blackness into a glowing

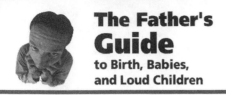

Chapter One

white image that was not a sunken ship, but clearly a baby in the early stages of development.

And, not just any baby. It was our baby.

Much like a photo booth at any self-respecting tourist destination, most ultrasound facilities are able to immediately print a picture of the ultrasound image of the baby for the parents to take home.

From the standpoint of an expectant father, who is not privy to the daily internal kicks and movement felt by the mother, holding that black-and-white glossy photo ultrasound photo is sort of the first tangible proof that the baby is on its way.

I remember it as a feeling of almost indescribable joy and not just because the baby already was much more photogenic than Leonardo DiCaprio.

In our case, we also were able to determine the gender of the baby through ultrasound. In this instance I am using the editorial "we," because the doctor was the first to know.

As soon as he knew, however, Karen also had to know. The thought of one other person on earth knowing that information when she did not would have driven her crazy. As a result, we left the office knowing that our first child was going to be a girl.

I immediately began visualizing the 12-foot-high fence around our yard to keep the boys away until she reached the age of, say, 35.

Let's Get Moving

For much of the pregnancy, the movements of the baby are felt internally only by the expectant mother. As the baby develops, however, the movements become more intense and eventually can be seen and felt by the outside world, quickly moving past cable TV as the family's No. 1 source of viewing pleasure.

Monitoring fetal movements is an inexact science, at best. And, as with other forms of comedy, timing is everything.

The mom-to-be will feel a healthy internal uppercut or karate kick and immediately say something like, "Quick! Come here. You can feel the baby move."

The male response typically is a heavy-sigh enhanced with an exaggerated rise from the couch to come and get a hands-on feel of the incredible moving stomach. Except, of course, it doesn't.

The minute the male hands touch the mother's abdomen, the baby retreats into perfect stillness. As soon as the male returns to the comfy confines of the couch, the baby kicks up a storm and maybe throws in a couple back flips.

Predictably, the entire follow-up process is repeated. Mom announces, dad sighs, baby stops kicking, dad feels nothing and sits back down, baby kicks again and mom announces. With any luck, it can evolve into an entire afternoon of affordable family fun.

Eventually, however, the expectant father will get lucky and feel one of the baby kicks or punches. Most men immediately take this as a sign that their child will be grow to be an NFL place kicker or possibly the star of a dubbed-language martial arts film.

Baby movements also can be triggered by loud noises. In our house, a stack of dropped dinner plates was good for a fair-sized abdominal jump. One of my coworkers, who was pregnant while I was writing this book, contributed a timely report on the effects of movie soundtracks on the baby. *Star Wars* was tolerable from a responsive movement standpoint, but *Spider Man* caused serious bouncing. Then again, maybe it was just more special effects.

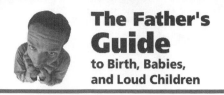
Chapter One

Surfing The Hormonal Waves

For those of you who quickly tire of the predictable, pregnancy is a period of constant change thanks to something called hormones. According to our faithful three-ring binder, an in-depth paragraph titled "Emotional Changes" says in tactful understatement that "mood swings are common." Not only are they common, they're frequent, random and totally unpredictable.

No two days are alike as the hormones vary, a personality pendulum swinging from one end of the emotional spectrum to the other. In fact, rarely does the emotional level remain constant from one hour to the next. Sometimes, you're lucky to get a consistent 10 minutes.

Anything and everything, and sometimes nothing at all, can trigger what is politely referred to as a mood swing, but can include anything from uncontrolled deep sobbing for no apparent reason to flat-out hormonal rage. At times there is little difference in the crisis of the minute. MY SHOE'S UNTIED!!! is accorded the same emotional importance as THE HOUSE IS ON FIRE!!

Pregnancy-related mood swings, while easy to acknowledge, are almost impossible for most guys to understand. After all, it's not their hormones that are on the rampage.

Actually, there probably is one, and only one, male who completely understood all the aspects of hormone-induced female mood swings. That would be actor Tony Perkins in his role as Norman Bates, wrapped in his mother's shawl screeching madly through the hallways of the Bates Motel in the movie, *Psycho*. The rest of us can only guess.

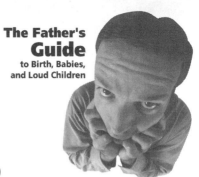

Chapter Two

You Can Help Now

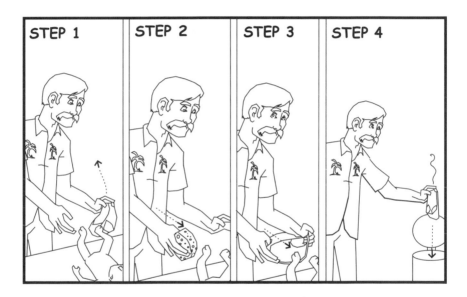

STEP 1   STEP 2   STEP 3   STEP 4

Reliable Delivery Person Wanted, Inquire Within

When it comes to performance, sports types tend to use the phrase "between the white lines," a statement that refers to how someone responds under actual game conditions regardless of practice habits.

In assessing my delivery room performance, I don't think I was ever the key to the lineup, but then again, I didn't have to be. Fortunately, Karen had a firm grasp on the pre-game planning and after that we thankfully were surrounded by people known as doctors and nurses.

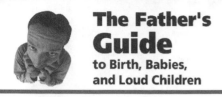
Chapter Two

In each of our three pregnancies, there were no at-home labor signals to indicate that it was time to rapidly head for the hospital. During each pregnancy, Karen had a blood-sugar condition known as gestational diabetes, which was carefully monitored, but resulted in extremely large babies. In each case, the doctor determined that induced labor at a specific time was necessary.

Most other couples we spoke with, however, received the "GO" signal at home in terms of regular and more frequent contractions and made the panicked, pedal-to-the-metal drive to the hospital.

The key to not giving birth in the center lane of rush-hour traffic is recognizing the signals of impending labor. This information is provided by the hospital or doctor who doesn't want to end up in rush-hour traffic any more than you do.

Just to confuse the issue is something known as false labor, also known as Braxton-Hicks Contractions, which apparently are named after a pair of renowned practical jokers. Braxton-Hicks Contractions resemble the real-labor contractions, but they are irregular and vary in length and intensity. Since you have no clue as to what is going on, it's best to defer to the expectant mother and just make sure the car has enough gas to get to the hospital when she says it's time.

During the birth of our first child, Karen was in mild labor from 8 a.m. to 5 p.m., followed by 12 hours of extremely hard labor, including three hours of pushing to try and get the baby out.

I had come off a fairly demanding work schedule and thought I was extremely tired. After watching Karen, I realized there is everyday work-related tired and then there is really, really, I'm-having-a-baby tired.

Once admitted to the maternity ward, the hospital staff ensured that the situation was constantly monitored from start to finish. As with much of the pregnancy, my role was mostly one of support, adjusting pillows, fetching water and pretending to know what I was doing when looking at the monitor printouts.

During the actual birth, it seemed like events were unfolding in slow motion, when in reality it was quite hectic.

As soon as the baby was born, the hospital staff settled into a much-practiced routine to efficiently and methodically take care of both mother and infant, keeping me safely out of the way.

Despite having used every last ounce of physical and emotional strength, Karen was cognizant enough to immediately ask, "Where is she?" followed by a hug that would last our baby a lifetime.

The Division of Labor

There is one bit of simple, yet sage, advice for the entire male population that will greatly increase chances for a long and prosperous life.

In mixed company, do not ever, under any circumstances or in any way, shape or form, refer to any part of the maternity process as "weenie labor."

This now-infamous quote is directly attributed to my long-ago college roommate, once known as Slobby Bobby, but now referred to as the more corporately correct, Rob. I meet him halfway and call him Bob.

Our long-standing friendship, firmly established on a foundation of rugby road trips and general collegiate weirdness, has now grown to include spouses and six, count 'em six, children ages 7 and under. Under the stressed-out-parents' portion of the misery loves sleepless company theory, our families have shared several vacations and weekend getaways. During one of the infrequent, uninterrupted, kids-are-napping, 2 1/2-minutes of adult conversation, the topic shifted to the birth of Bob and his wife, Shelli's, second child, Evan.

The details are somewhat hazy, but the gist of the story, I think, was that Evan apparently had not given them much advance warning about his desire to join the world. As part of his delivery room role, Bob was in charge of monitoring the contraction print-out, offering medically unsubstantiated, yet supportive, comments like, "That wasn't a very big one," and, "Oops, here comes a really big one."

As the process gathered momentum, the time frame for administering an epidural somehow jumped directly from "it's too early," to "sorry, it's, too late."

While explaining to us how the window of pain-relief opportunity had slammed shut, Bob said something about the contraction sheet showing that Shelli had not been in actual labor-labor, but that it was more like, well, you know, "weenie labor."

The simultaneous response from every female in the room was immediate and deafening.

HOW WOULD YOU KNOW!!!

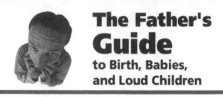

Chapter Two

Bob immediately began the verbal backpedaling, but to no avail. Never had one tennis-shoe encased foot been jammed so far down one throat. While the phrase "weenie labor" may never be included in medical textbooks, the point is clear and unarguable. When it comes to maternity ward bragging rights, membership in this labor union is clearly restricted.

Males need not apply. For one simple reason. They can't.

Throughout the maternity process, men can participate and support, but no matter how much they are involved, in the end they are reduced to the role of spectator, although one with a really good seat.

Even male doctors, in fact especially male doctors, are not immune from the division of labor.

After much research and careful deliberation, my wife settled on a wonderful female doctor with whom she felt both comfortable and confident.

As we approached the due date, our regular doctor informed us that there was a chance she would be out of town, but there was a reliable and experienced doctor, albeit a male one, ready as a backup.

One of our delivery-room nurses reassuringly said something about reserve Dr. So-and-so having delivered hundreds of babies. Karen's response was that good old male Dr. So-and-so might have caught a bunch of newborn babies, but he had never actually delivered one.

As difficult as it may be, there are many, many other instances where men should simply be seen and not heard throughout the duration of pregnancy.

Recently on a televised panel discussion, another male medical expert foolishly compared the pain of some sort of intestinal problem to that of labor. Several million TV-watching mothers shouted at their sets in unison, HOW WOULD YOU KNOW!!! Dozens of others undoubtedly bounced their remotes off his smug TV forehead.

Although it is politically correct and baby boomer trendy for men to use the phrase "We're pregnant," I would strongly urge that most males silently file this one away in their drawer full of unused stupid.

The reason, I hope, is painfully obvious.

From the female point of view, if "we" are so pregnant, how come only one of us is throwing up, gaining weight, not sleeping and battling a more-than-occasional hormone surge. Feel free to jump in at any time and share the workload, big guy.

Nope, in some instances it is simply better to keep your mouth shut and recognize a good biological deal when you see one. After that, there is only one thing to remember. There is no such thing as weenie labor. Unless you like the taste of tennis shoes.

Name That Name

The quest for the perfect name is the parental equivalent of the Holy Grail, a tireless search for the moniker that will serve as a foolproof stepping stone to greatness.

No alphabetical stone is left unturned, no source left untapped when it comes to finding the name that most parents believe will launch their children on the path to lifelong success.

Many a sleepless night is spent as prospective parents agonize over the selection they believe is destined to appear in conjunction with such phrases as CEO, senator, all-star, Nobel prize winner or, at the very least, lucky Lotto ticket holder.

In reality, of course, the process of separating every Tom, Dick and Harry from every Tom, Dick and Harry is at best a well-intentioned crapshoot. A roll of the naming dice has just as much chance of producing a future police blotter entrant as it does a member of Congress, although the two now seem to frequently overlap.

Previous parental naming disasters have narrowed the field, eliminating such middle-name miscues as John Wilkes or Lee Harvey. Among biblical choices, Judas does not exactly rank right up there with Matthew, Mark, Luke and John.

Change, in the form of industrialization, urbanization and MTV, has done away with entire generations of once-popular names. Elementary school classrooms are no longer filled with Elmers, Oscars or Floyds pulling the pigtails of an Edna, Ethel, Blanch or Gladys.

By the same token, it's hard to picture a bunch of Kaitlyns, Ashleys, Justins and Brandons someday locked in a cut-throat game of hearts in a beachside retirement home.

Image also has taken its toll on some names.

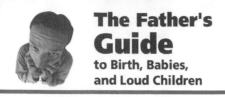

Chapter Two

In World War I, the largest piece of artillery was nicknamed "Big Bertha." The point was further hammered home sometime in the early '70s thanks to a band known as the Jimmy Castor Bunch, whose song "Troglodyte" included a flattering line that went something like, "Bertha, Bertha Butt. She was one of the Butt sisters."

It will be a long, long time before the world sees a fashion model named Bertha.

For similar reasons, I've always thought that if we named one of our children, Eb, we might as well just go ahead and sew the patch on the Texaco shirt. Of course, since I can't change a spark plug, this might not be such a bad thing.

Some parents draw their naming inspiration from somewhat unusual sources. According to basketball lore and many barroom wagers, basketball Hall of Famer Elgin Baylor was so-named after his father looked down at his Elgin watch in the waiting room. None of our children ever will be named Rolex.

In my own family, I have been told (jokingly, I hope) that one of the possibilities my dad was considering for me was Luten Oxel. I have no idea where this came from or what it could possibly mean, although if my mother hadn't stepped in, my wife says my magazine column would be called "Bachelor's 'Hood" instead of "Father's 'Hood."

To help beleaguered parents arrive at the perfect name, the point-of-purchase folks have stocked supermarket checkout aisles with a variety of baby name books. For less than the cost of a *National Enquirer*, those waiting to pay for groceries can get a 100-page head start on the process, including the origin and meaning of each name.

In the interest of journalistic research, I picked up a copy that promised "hundreds of useful tips."

According to this source, Ace is still an option for male children, especially for those families looking to start their own outlaw motorcycle gang. The meaning for Dennis is listed as "wild and crazy, from Dionysus, the god of food and wine." This explains the Rodman family's decision.

The source of some names is hard to pinpoint. For example, in Middle English, Farrah stems from "beautiful one," while in Arabic, it means "wild donkey." This may be a contributing factor to the lack of Ms. Fawcett film festivals in the Middle East.

In our house, rather than rely on a book or the psychic hotline, we used a much more scientific formula for determining name acceptability.

Ready? On the count of three...

Hayley, Hayley bo bayley banana fana fo fayley me my mo mayley, Hayley.

Now, let's try Tyler.

Tyler, Tyler bo byler banana fana fo fyler me my mo myler, Tyler.

How 'bout Colin?

Colin, Colin bo bolin banana fana fo folin me my mo molin, Colin.

They sounded good to us. Now, bring on those lucky Lotto tickets.

The Long Lost World Of Sleep

A recent survey by some well-rested study group indicates that something like 80 percent of adult Americans do not get enough sleep.

These are called parents.

And, you do not need a government grant to know that the remaining 20 percent obviously do not have children, do not know people that have children, or do not live within two zip codes of people that have children.

The heartwarming phrase, "sleeping like a baby," is not only an oxymoron, it's almost non-existent. When it comes to sleep, infants and toddlers are not the voices of experience, they are the non-stop, top-of-the-lung chorus of second-hand insomnia.

According to encyclopedic research (done in conjunction with the Nite Owl movie and six pots of French Roast), "normal periods of sleep range from six to nine hours each night, with seven and a half hours being the average."

That certainly was the case in our three-child household. Seven and a half hours of total sleep, divided almost equally among the five bleary-eyed occupants.

Of course, the same article says "a newborn may sleep as much as 16 hours a day in intermittent periods, or naps, and a 2-year-old may sleep from nine to 12 hours." This purveyor of infant gospel (who may or may not have gone on to write "Face of Jesus Appears in Corn Flakes Bowl" stories for supermarket tabloids) obviously has never

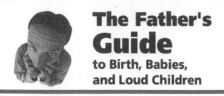
Chapter Two

come face to red-screaming-face at 2 a.m., 4 a.m. or any other wide-awake a.m.

And, the ability of one child to keep an entire household awake for months at a time pales in comparison to the full-volume tandem ability of a pair of non-sleepers. Even if one of the two is a good sleeper, there is some sort of obligation among those with footy pajamas requiring both to form a world championship tag team designed to keep their punch-drunk parents on the ropes of sleeplessness. It's a simple prearranged plan where one child cries until exhaustion sets in, thereby automatically waking child No. 2, who takes over the crying chores, giving child No. 1 plenty of time to rest up for the next round of no rest.

When both kids finally pass out, one or both parents then cry from exhaustion. This is the now-popular cry-it-out theory.

Despite the efforts of the best scientific minds in the world, no one knows for sure why some babies sleep, well, like babies, while others (ours) spent more time awake at night than Dracula.

In the first year, however, it generally is conceded that all 365 consecutive sleepless nights are simply the result of gas.

A 12-pack of Leinenkugel's beer and four bowls of chili could not generate as much gas as your standard, everyday throw-most-of-it-on-the-floor jar of baby food. And, the actual B-movie sounding "Attack of the Giant Gas Bubble" directly coincides with the shutting of parental eyelids.

Once verbal ability sets in, no 2-year-old says, "I have gas," but there is no shortage of reasons for a toddler's inability to sleep.

"I'm hot, I'm cold, I'm hungry, I'm thirsty, I have a tummy ache, I don't have a tummy ache, I'm wet, Are you asleep?" all are part of the non-stop running commentary.

Frank Sinatra never worked a Las Vegas microphone as well as Hayley, Tyler and Colin worked the business end of a baby monitor.

Because identifying a problem is not necessarily the same as solving it, my late-night research also turned up the following under the heading "Sleep Deprivation" – "When humans are totally deprived of sleep for several days, they may experience irritability, blurred vision, slurred speech, memory lapses and confusion."

I have noticed some of that when writing this book where I tend to repeat myself sometimes in this book and many of the sentences do not make a whole lot of sense about sleep sometimes not late at night when I'm a parent writing this parenting book about parents.

Then again, maybe I'm just tired.

Staying Abreast Of The Situation

When it comes to needs, most newborns have their priorities straight. From the get-go, it's time to eat. In some instances, this means breastfeeding, while others opt for bottle-fed formula. A myriad of factors enter into the decision. Sometimes it based on doctor's advice while other times it's simply a matter of personal preference. In some instances, such as if or when the new mother returns to work, it's simply based on practicality.

Karen opted to breastfeed each of our children which from a father's standpoint is as good as it gets because once again, you avoid all the work based on gender.

Every two or three hours for a period of almost three years, Karen and the kids were attached, well not at the hip, but you get the picture. Although this regimen somewhat hampered her social life, Karen did manage to squeeze in one outing with some lifelong friends. To make sure that everything was covered at home, meaning that even I couldn't mess it up, she used a breast pump to fill a couple bottles with breast milk in case the baby rang the dinner bell while Karen was gone.

When filling the bottles seemed to take longer than expected, I went upstairs to check on her. As I climbed the stairs, I began to hear what, to me, sounded like the rhythmic up-and-down droning of a small jet ski engine. Apparently, the demands of new motherhood had taken it's toll. Karen was sound asleep in the recliner, breast pump attached and humming merrily away as what appeared to be a water-fall of milk spilled over the side of the bottle and onto the floor below. She can laugh about it now. Sort of. Well, once in a while.

On rare occasions, we augmented the breastfeeding with formula. Although I carefully read and re-read the instructions on the side of the container, there was nothing in writing that indicated I could not participate.

We did learn one concrete lesson about formula feeding, as did several people seated around us. We were flying home from a family

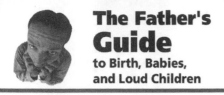
vacation (i.e., staying for free with relatives), when Karen realized we did not have any prepared baby bottles of formula. Apparently, sucking on a baby bottle during take-off and landing helps infants equalize the pressure in their ears, somewhat reducing the chance of an hour-long, uncontrollable crying outburst.

Although we had a small amount of formula powder, we had nothing to mix it with until Karen discovered the can of sparkling water in the darkest reaches of the diaper bag.

She mixed the formula and carbonated water according to the directions, gave it a quick shake and BOOOOM!!! It was like a formula bomb exploded. Obviously, there was some sort of reaction between the formula and the canned water. The people around us, especially those within the spatter zone, did not find it nearly as humorous as we did.

The Times They Are A-Changin'

I'm guessing that, like might most men, you paid strict attention to each and every pregnancy-related detail of the prenatal classes. But, in case your mind wandered off on a leisurely mental stroll to anywhere but the classroom, reality has a way of quickly filling in the academic gaps.

And nothing is more of an instant refresher course than diaper changing, where classroom theory immediately gives way to practical application.

One of the first things that makes itself evident in the household of the newborn is the fact that babies and infants are glorified food processors, cradle-sized alchemists capable of turning minuscule amounts of breast milk and formula into gallons of diaper-filling lava.

From day one, their digestive track is always on and continuously set to operate at high speed, churning away 24 hours a day, 7 days a week, 365 days a year.

The end result is immediately noticeable. There is no guesswork involved. When it comes to diaper-changing time, the nose knows.

Unlike such things as breast-feeding, where participation is limited by nature, diaper changing is one of those rare, gender-free obligations where men can, and should, share equally in the enjoyment.

You Can Help Now

Mike Carter, a songwriting friend from Oklahoma and the father of two young children, lyrically captured the spirit of fatherly participation in the span of two minutes and 48 seconds with a tune called, "Real Dads Do Diapers."

The first verse and the chorus go like this:

"Some dads do dishes, and others cook and clean,
And there's a few who know how to use a washing machine.
Well fatherhood's a never-ending responsibility,
From taking out the trash to the vasectomy.
Real dads do diapers, they get up at 3 a.m.
To rock and burp and doctor that brand-new little kid
And real dads aren't afraid of a little poop or puke or pee
Real dads do diapers and they do 'em in their sleep."

Mike is not a famous songwriter, just a very perceptive one.

In many instances, olfactory sense determines who mans the changing table. Those with an extremely sensitive and highly developed sense of smell often are able to catch a preliminary whiff of things to come, thereby enabling them to make a quick exit, leaving the slow-to-smell to savor another round of hands-on parenting experience.

At times, even a keen sense of hearing can be a parental asset. For example, if you hear what appears to be a small corporate jet taking off, yet you live nowhere near an airport, it is a good idea to give the nearest diaper at least a cursory inspection.

For me personally, diaper changing was something that I not only didn't mind doing, it was something I could do with a relative amount of confidence.

The process of diaper changing does not have a gray area of unknown. It is not like trying to diagnose a cold, fever or the flu, along with the consequential pressure of a blown call. It does not have the societal stress of wardrobe matching and color coordination.

It is a simple, straightforward, step-by-step procedure. Off, clean, on, dispose. A one-bottom latrine detail. Even someone beset with allergies can usually hold their breath long enough to complete the task.

The key to successful diaper changing is quickness and the key to quickness is the wardrobe.

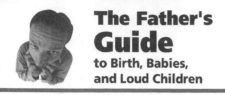
Chapter Two

Newborns tend to lay around in sack-like dressing gowns, allowing easy access for diaper changing. You just push the sack up above their waist, do the quick-change routine, wash your hands, and there's still enough time to hit the refrigerator before the end of the commercial.

Once pants come in to play, however, it is a different matter entirely. Everything revolves around snaps. A series of snaps up one inside seam, across the crotch and down the other seam provides an easy-opening maintenance hatch for diaper duty. In many instances the diaper also is covered by the proverbial "onesie," an undershirt that snaps at the crotch, but that is easily handled by even the most fumble fingered of fathers.

Pants without snaps present a myriad of problems. For one thing, they have to be pulled all the way down, if not completely off, to begin the changing process. If the pants have to be removed, they invariably do not fit over the shoes. As such, the shoes have to come off, then the pants, thereby increasing the squirm factor.

Trust me as the voice of experience on this one. The worst possible outfit for diaper changing is bib overalls with snap-free legs; a sweater or sweatshirt worn over the straps of the bibs; and a pair of cute, but impossible to tie, miniature hiking boots.

Minutes quickly become hours when trying to unassemble and reassemble this outfit, not to mention the risk of dizziness through oxygen deprivation after holding your breath beyond the recommended safety limits.

Regardless of the wardrobe, once the diaper is changed, the entire process is, of course, repeated in reverse. You will then have anywhere from three minutes to an hour before having to do it again.

Once the onesie is unsnapped, the actual changing becomes a one-handed job. If the changee is lying on his or her back, one adult hand holds both ankles while the other hand does all the dirty work.

Unsuspecting parents usually only make the mistake of letting go of the ankles one time. The spattering effect of a kicking infant with the leg power of an NFL field-goal kicker is a tremendous teaching tool.

You Can Help Now

When it comes to the diapers themselves, there are basically two kinds, disposable and cloth, also known as the old-fashioned kind.

Disposable diapers are exactly what they claim to be. Once used, they are simply thrown away. Much like the dilemma surrounding the disposal of toxic waste, however, exactly where the diapers are thrown away is a tough call.

At the risk of a blatant product endorsement, I would highly recommend a gizmo known as the Diaper Genie. It's basically a plastic canister with a closable lid and loaded inside with a replaceable roll of plastic wrap. The used diaper is placed inside the Diaper Genie, the top of which is then given a spin. The twisting motion seals the diaper (and hopefully its odor) inside the plastic wrap, much like the casing on a sausage. The process is repeated for each successive diaper, creating a sealed-in chain of diaper links.

When the Diaper Genie canister is full, the hinged bottom opens allowing the entire chain to be dropped into a plastic bag. The whole bag can then be carried outside to the garbage cans to the delight of the guys who pick up the trash on hot days.

A sports writing friend of mine who for years has covered losing major league baseball teams for the *Milwaukee Journal Sentinel* and is the father of an 18-month-old calls the Diaper Genie, "the greatest invention since the remote." By press box standards, that is heady praise, indeed.

There are about six gazillion different kinds of disposable diapers on the market of varying shapes, styles and styles. It is almost impossible not to find the kind appropriate for you. In most instances, it's simply a matter of personal choice, although size is critical.

Too big and the diapers leak around the edges. Too small and the pressure results in a geyser-like spray, usually up the middle of the back.

From what we were able to determine, disposable diapers come in three price ranges. Expensive, more expensive and who is your co-signer?

We were extremely fortunate during Hayley's infancy to have a friend who worked at a paper mill in the diaper division. One of his perks was the ability to purchase gigantic cases of diapers at an overwhelming employee discount.

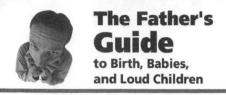
Chapter Two

He came to our house one Thanksgiving for dinner and unloaded what appeared to be a small refrigerator from his Jeep. Instead of an office-sized Frigidaire, the box held hundreds of disposable diapers. It was the ultimate gift for a family on an hourly changing schedule.

Unfortunately, word of this veritable gold mine soon filtered out amongst those with small children and his social calendar filled up for the next several decades.

Because we wimped out under the guise of convenience and used disposable diapers and wipes, I actually know very little about cloth diapers except that they serve the same purpose, but it takes an engineering degree from MIT to make them stay on. They also have to be laundered. The last thing we ever needed in our house was more laundry.

There also are diaper services that will deliver, pickup and launder your diapers. We have another friend who used one of these services. She mentioned the phrase "plastic pants" and also used the word "leaking" several times when describing her experience. Diaper services can be found in the local Yellow Pages and I'm sure they would appreciate the chance to give you a more detailed description of what they have to offer.

Many doctors say that the parental calls regarding such things as the common cold and flu pale in comparison to the number of inquiries regarding infant and toddler bowel movements.

My sister's pediatrician says the majority of calls received by his office involve such phrases as "too hard, too soft, too runny, too yellow and not yellow enough."

He has one simple pediatric philosophy concerning this particular occurrence. "Americans are entirely too preoccupied with bowel movements. If it happens, good. If it hasn't, it will."

Standing Up For Stand-Ups

The switch from the comfort of diapers changed by others to taking responsibility for your own actions is a major change and frequently not an easy one.

For little girls, the switch from potty-chair to full-size toilet simply means a bigger seat. Little boys, on the other hand, literally have to aim to change.

Rather than face the cold-plastic prospect of plopping on to a potty chair, our middle son, Tyler, decided to take a stand in the battle to end all diapers.

Like a 3-foot-tall John Wayne, he staunchly decided to stand on his own two feet in the definitive move from diaper-wearing toddler to underwear-clad little boy.

From his perspective, sitting down on the job was just not going to happen.

We're not quite sure if the proverbial potty training battle was tougher that time around due to the difference in gender, apathy or just plain stubbornness.

When Hayley decided to make the move from diapers, her mind was made up. One day diaper, the next day underwear. And, by the way, dad, I need some new underwear to match my outfits. Really expensive underwear. And, lots of it.

Tyler, on the other hand, dashed past his third birthday with little inclination toward shedding his cloth-like, ultra-absorbent, super-stretch, Velcro-attached, no-marketing-phrase-left-unturned diaper. He seemed quite content to amble through life with the bulging behind of a bunched-up diaper. Visions of his eventual first job interview were not encouraging.

The addition of our third child, Colin, who received the air-freshening attention associated with 47 daily diaper changings, did not make Tyler's task any easier. Several times Tyler was stranded atop the potty chair while Colin was being changed, oops, changed, oops, and changed again. From Tyler's perspective, it was easy to see who was getting the short end of the changing stick.

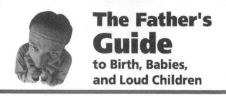
Chapter Two

From a male standpoint, I tried to convince Tyler of some of the advantages of doing away with his diapers. This convincing was usually done out of the earshot of mom.

I told him, for example, that when nature calls, moms, sisters and aunts usually have to rely on call-waiting, driving miles out of the way for a clean, well-lit, sanitized, germ-free, dust-proof, hermetically-sealed restroom. With a big lock.

Guys can simply turn to any bush except George W.

I also may have alluded to the perfect penmanship developed through the mid-winter use of a previously pristine snow bank (not from personal experience, of course) as well as the advantages of digesting an entire sports section in the chapel-like solitude of a well-bolted men's room.

One Wisconsin songwriter perfectly captured this male ritual in a heartfelt ditty titled, "Every Man," which contains the line "every man needs a bathroom with a fan, 'cause every man likes to read while on the can."

It's almost embarrassing how many compact discs he sold because of that one song to aficionados of classical music and admirers of fine art. Cashing those checks may be the ultimate in bathroom humor.

Despite my heroic tales of men in the wild and the suggestion of song, the best motivator for toilet training was the good old-fashioned urinal, or, stand-ups, as Tyler called them.

From his point of view, there was nothing easier than waddling up to a stand-up and taking care of business. There was no struggling climb to the top of a too-high toilet, no prospect of an icy, unintentional dip through a too-wide opening.

In a relatively short period of time, Tyler became an authority on restrooms, analyzing each and every piece of porcelain with the skeptical eye of a hard-to-please plumbing inspector. He brazenly barged into every men's room, quickly scanned the furnishings and gave his top-of-the-lung report.

NO STAND UPS!! or ONLY ONE SIT-DOWN!! followed by some in-depth accounting of cleanliness, smell and current occupancy. This investigative reporting always was appreciated by nearby restaurant patrons hovering in mid-forkful.

Soon after Colin's arrival, we talked with an architect about remodeling our house. Tyler lobbied strongly that any remodeled bathrooms include those "stand-ups," especially since Colin also was a little boy.

In no uncertain terms, Karen vetoed that suggestion.

You Can Help Now

With the prospects of our installing home-based urinals standing solidly between none and absolutely not, Tyler finally ascended to the next level with the fixtures at hand. That same day, he received his official graduation announcement from Hayley.

"Tyler, put the seat down!"

Welcome to the real world.

A Fluid Situation

Aside from the difficulties of toilet training, everything else in our household operation is remarkably fluid. Unbelievably fluid. Astonishingly fluid. Astoundingly, stupendously, soaked-up-to-our-whatever in fluid.

Since our first child arrived on the scene, there has not been one single, solitary day where something was not spilled, spattered, sprayed or splashed. Since that day, every square inch of our humble abode has been saturated from wall to wall and floor to ceiling, then drip-by-drip to the floor below.

After every meal, the kitchen resembles the aftermath of an *Animal House* food fight. Plumbing and appliances that hummed merrily along in the pre-children era now leak like 40-year-old rowboats. Drains are stopped up by nothing more than a dirty look. Potty training takes place anywhere but the potty. In our house, a puddle jumper is not a small airplane.

To ensure that the continuing string of household disasters stays at least two cluttered rooms ahead of the exasperated two-person clean-up crew, our children are chronologically spaced for maximum spillage.

As of this morning's trail of breakfast crumbs, Hayley was seven, Tyler six and Colin three. We are the quintessential family-sized pack of Instant Mess – just add liquid.

Even our dog, Drysdale, (known, but not officially recognized, as the world's dumbest dog) has gotten into the act. Everything makes him throw up. Dry dog food, canned dog food, gourmet dog food, dust, loud noises and, apparently, gulps of fresh air all trigger some sort of middle-of-the-night hacking fest with the end result usually placed strategically along what is best described as a barefoot path. His barf is definitely worse than his bite.

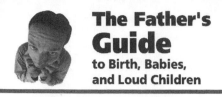
Chapter Two

When it comes to mess making as an art form, the kitchen is a rainbow-colored palette of potential. Placing squeeze bottles in the hands of children is like putting a brush in the hands of Picasso. There is nothing like a healthy, two-handed squirt of ketchup or mustard to complement most wardrobes.

Because Hayley, Tyler and Colin approach every meal with the motto, "we aim to stain," color coordination is important. Chocolate is never spilled on brown pants. Tomato soup is wasted on a red skirt. Blueberries on blue jeans? Heck, you might as well not spill anything at all.

One of the most interesting phenomena of childhood dining is the invisible milk glass. While standing rock solid in full view of all adults, most milk glasses apparently cannot be seen by children who attempt to reach right through them while grabbing for something else.

Got Milk?

Yes, in a puddle on the floor, at least once a day.

Early physics lessons also are a matter of spillage. Today's solid Popsicle is tomorrow's liquid puddle, which soon becomes forever's red stain. We put the pillow over that part of the couch.

As makers of movies with sophomoric humor have discovered (or so I've heard), bathroom humor generates an easy laugh. During the diaper phase, as in most good slapstick routines, timing is everything.

Seldom is a diaper changed at a leisurely pace one hour before a scheduled departure for anywhere. Studies have shown that the bodily functions of most infants are directly tied to the opening of a car door.

For true comedic effect, baby boys have the added advantage of what is known as "the arc." In the split second between removal of the old diaper and placement of the new one, most baby boys respond to pressure with pressure. A true master will not only dampen the new diaper, but also much of the surrounding area. At his best, Colin has soaked a fresh set of bedding, his new outfit, the fresh clothes of the person doing the changing, a folded pile of laundry and the open pages of an overdue library book.

In family lore, this is known as the Arc de Triomphe.

I had one more example of family disaster to recount, but I'm actually being served lunch at my desk by Hayley and Tyler. Judging by the trail on the carpet behind them, I think we're having soup.

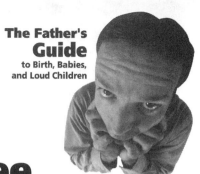

Chapter Three

Keeping Up Appearances

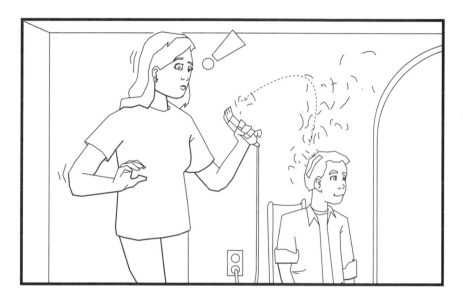

Dressed For Distress

My usual journalistic disdain for appropriate attire has served me well in many a major-league press box. Unfortunately, it also has left me pitifully unprepared for the daily rigors of that fast-growing indoor sport known as infant dressing.

On most days, my own unimaginative wardrobe consists of faded jeans, tennis shoes and a T-shirt that usually says something catchy like, "Jack Ingram and the Beat-Up Ford Band." The entire outfit requires one snap, takes seven seconds to complete and eliminates the prospect of mismatched polyester plaids.

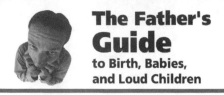
Chapter Three

The miniature brand-name world of Carter's, Baby B'Gosh and Something-Trendy-And-Expensive-For-Kids, however, is an entirely different matter, an unnerving morning ritual of tugging and twisting, pulling and prodding, all in the name of fashion while covering a diaper the size of Rhode Island.

From socks to sweaters, pants to pullovers, jumpers to jackets, the color-coordinated intricacies of toddler-wear defy logic and adult fingers. Snaps that march logically up pant legs like an orderly game of connect-the-dots, suddenly disintegrate into an unsolvable corduroy puzzle – a Rubik's cube of the crotch.

I suspect some demented designers, whose own parents probably refused to seek the necessary co-signers for a pair of Baby Nike's, simply put an extra snap on one side of their outfits as a fiendish measure of revenge.

In many instances, these seemingly harmless pieces of clothing are almost symmetrical. Fronts look like backs, tops look like bottoms and does this button connect here, here or here?

Although my own wardrobe may lack splendor, it is simplistically consistent. For example, the little half-inch orange cloth vertical tag that simply says "Levis" is always reassuringly found on the right pocket of my continually expanding backside. Always has been, always will be.

Not so with Baby-Something-Or-Others, I discovered. During one of my well-intentioned first-year attempts, I carefully and caringly dressed Hayley, applying to her little blue jeans the time-tested Levis approach of tag in the back.

The pink tag should have been a clue, but it wasn't until the middle of the party that another sharp-eyed parent loudly pointed out how cute it was that, "her pants are on backwards." I'm sure the embarrassment eventually will be overcome with several thousand dollars worth of therapy and a compensated appearance on Jerry Springer.

Baby sleeves are another great mystery of the universe. How can an eight-inch arm completely disappear in a seven-inch sleeve? Unshakable certainties such as physics and gravity do not apply to the real-life laws of turtlenecks under the size of 2-T.

Keeping Up Appearances

I've saved the smallest for last. Baby socks are, without a doubt, the source of roughly half the country's problems. When washed, they separate to different zip codes. When dried, they curl into colored balls the size of marbles and attach themselves to the inside of an adult pant leg, eventually reappearing out of dad's cuff in the grocery store check-out line.

Actually attempting to put socks on a baby's foot is like to trying to stuff a hamster in a sausage casing. The same foot that goes stubbornly rigid when being coaxed into a shoe, turns instantly to Jell-O at the merest touch of a sock. If by some miracle you actually get both feet covered, the automatic sock ejectors kick in. With no conspicuous motion, first one sock, then the other is unceremoniously jettisoned, usually in public and usually over a puddle.

Baby shoes actually last as long as advertised, mostly because they are outgrown an hour after purchase. Even the most active baby has a tough time destroying a pair of shoes in that initial hour. As such, we have storage boxes full of various-sized hand-me-down shoes in a wide range of colors. Many a fun family afternoon has been spent sifting through boxes of kid shoes, hoping to find a matching pair to hand down to the next in line. It's sort of like the shoe version of Crazy 8s, except it takes just one pair to win. On particularly behind-schedule days where mom is not around to help with the finer points, it has not been unusual for the youngest to be wearing one blue sneaker and one white sneaker while accompanying dad on the errand of the day.

Despite my own ineptitude, however, the one thing that is quite clear is that, in the end, brand names matter little. The packaging pales in comparison to the package. It just so happens that ours always have been wrapped in stuff like "Jack Ingram and the Beat-Up Ford Band" T-shirts.

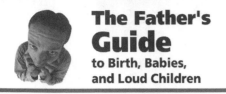

Chapter Three

Hair Today, Gone Tomorrow

From a father's standpoint, hair care may be even more difficult to master than the daily wardrobe. Based on my own comb-free, throw-on-a-ballcap approach to hair care, Karen has assumed all duties in that area, especially with Hayley.

From a very young age, Hayley and Karen have covered the gamut of daily options – ponytail, side ponytails, pigtails, braids, French braids, buns and who knows what else.

The boys, on the other hand, can usually be readied with a wet brush and a straight part. I can almost handle that. If not, we have kid-sized ballcaps.

But even in the relatively uneventful world of kids' hair, there are bad hair days and, then again, there are bad hair days.

Your average run-of-the-mill, just another day in the press box bad hair day usually involves nothing more than a routine case of hat head, pillow head or sleepless-parent-of-three-children head.

On one memorable occasion in our house, the other end of the tonsorial spectrum was Hayley hair. Or, more appropriately, the lack of it.

Our first experience with gender-based hair care occurred when Hayley was three years old. When I left on a weekend music trip, she was the possessor of the proverbial long, blond flowing locks, the daily mother-and-daughter playground of piggies, ponies, braids and barrettes.

One from-the-road phone call later, however, and it was obvious that the hair world at home had been turned upside down. Although I received the story second-hand over several hundred miles of long distance telephone wire, the gist of the disaster was readily apparent.

With a couple clicks of rounded safety scissors, Hayley had hacked a handful of randomly selected hunks of hair from her bumper blond crop and then carefully stashed it in the pockets of her dress.

Karen was talking on the telephone with one of her sisters when Hayley appeared around the corner with her new 'do. Karen's shocked silence drew an immediate "What's wrong?" from Aunt Leslie's end of the phone conversation.

Keeping Up Appearances

Hayley was extremely proud of her first attempt at haircutting until she saw the look on Karen's face, which then triggered an avalanche of unstoppable sobbing.

The stage-whispered description that I received over the telephone was basically that Hayley had, indeed, done a bit of self-barbering, trimming her bangs almost to the hairline, whacking one side up over the ear and taking random chunks out of the back.

For some reason, all I could picture was a three-foot-tall Cyndi Lauper.

(As part of today's pop music history lesson, the aforementioned Ms. Lauper was a colorful New Wave singer noted for the early '80s classic song, "Girls Just Want To Have Fun." Her stage persona included avant-garde outfits, wild haircuts – including one side of her head shaved – and multi-colored hairdos. A decade later, basketball player-turned-publicity hound Dennis Rodman became the new Cyndi Lauper.)

Anyway, Hayley eventually got on the phone and said in a trembling voice, "I cut my hair," which was again followed by an avalanche of sobbing.

I finally calmed her down with a lengthy tale of how, as a little boy, I also had cut my own hair and it eventually grew back (only to fall out again some 35 years later, although that is another story.)

My hair-cutting tale was a bit of the proverbial white lie, designed to stem the flood of long-distance tears. My own childhood hair disaster actually involved a hideous product known as Butch Wax, a thick, pink tar-like substance that was gobbed onto a juvenile head for so-called grooming purposes. Running a comb through Butch Wax-laden hair actually left grooves across your head, much like rake marks in a sand trap. Magazine ads picturing suave, Butch Wax-using guys attracting scads of women were accurate only if you substituted bumblebees for females.

Anyway, at some point, my grade school haircut evolved from the basic, marine-style buzz cut to the trendier flattop, held in place, of course, by an adult-supervised application of Butch Wax. Not wanting to miss a moment in my ascension up the second grade ladder of hip haircuts, I got up long before dawn to slather the Butch Wax across my new flattop.

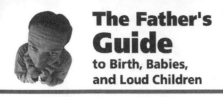

Chapter Three

Boy, did I slather. My entire head was one pink sticky ball. It looked like someone had blown a giant bubble-gum bubble and stuck it atop my shoulders. Three weeks and several dozen varieties of shampoo later, we were still washing Butch Wax remains out of my hair. (In fact, to this day, I swear there's a slight pinkish tint on my pillow after a hot, humid night.)

The result of the Butch Wax fiasco was the end of the great flattop experiment and a return to the relative maintenance-free safety of the crewcut.

By the time I returned home from my musical weekend, Hayley had been zipped over to a nearby beauty parlor for a bit of shaping, trimming and general camouflage. All in all, it didn't look too bad. At least it wasn't pink.

M Marks The Spot

While Hayley was responsible for her own hair disaster, Tyler had help in the form of Karen's first attempt at home barbering. A quick glimpse at the back of Tyler's recently trimmed head after that first effort brought back images of a long-ago, hard-learned lesson: Few things in the world of kiddom attract attention and corresponding ridicule like home barbering.

As a buzz cut battered, no-Beatles'-haircuts-allowed veteran of my dad's do-it-yourself styling efforts, I had taken the parental vow of never, ever attempting to trim a single hair on the head of any of our children.

As a constant reminder, a cupboard in our downstairs bathroom still contains my dad's old hair clippers, the destructive power nestled at the ready in the original, now faded, red, white and blue box that cheerily proclaimed on its side, "Be A Happy Home Barber."

Nothing was ever said about the unhappy barberee.

As such, I am pictured in most old family photos wearing a baseball cap, football helmet or Tupperware bowl, along with the perpetual frown of the involuntarily trimmed.

If I was willing to shell out several thousand dollars for a professional opinion, I'm sure my continuing aversion to hair clippers would be diagnosed as some sort of post-traumatic stress syndrome and a welcome topic on the TV talk show circuit.

Keeping Up Appearances

Having never viewed firsthand the after-effects of a basic training barber's chair, Karen had no such reservations about taking the proverbial bit off Tyler's top.

To that end, Karen and the kids returned from a shopping trip with a sparkling new hair clipper, complete with the how-to video explaining "Home Haircutting With Wahl." According to the marketing material, Wahl, whomever he is, "makes it easy."

The video, which also includes Spanish subtitles, promised a step-by-step guide to a perfect cut, including, but not limited to, tips on clipper use and care; contemporary cuts; buzz cuts; flattops; the fade and longer hairstyles.

As an extra added bonus, the video packaging literally exclaimed in bold letters, "New! Now includes instructions for Wahl's exclusive 1-1/2 inch guide and 5-position combs." Like an eager-to-learn class of barber college freshmen, Karen and the kids plopped down in front of the small kitchen TV to absorb the varied and valuable techniques of home hairstyling.

True to its word, the video began with the chirpy-voiced encouragement that, Wahl, did indeed, make it easy. Or, for those reading the bottom of the screen, "Con Wahl, todo es mas facil!"

Using a series of drawings of human heads, reminiscent of TV documentaries on presidential assassinations, home haircutting was quickly and expertly explained in a series of logical steps.

The video then progressed through a series of techniques and examples using a group of young models who sit perfectly still through a variety of scalpel attacks.

The end result was, of course, an entire group of freshly trimmed, immaculately coiffed, smiling models whose mere appearance testified to the joys of home hairstyling.

Bolstered by Wahl's video reassurance and armed with the confidence of an avid watcher of home remodeling TV programs, Karen fired up the trusty Wahl Homepro Adjustable to give Tyler his first do-it-yourself home haircut.

I wandered in to the kitchen in time to find Karen hovering around a partially trimmed Tyler, clutching the still-smoking weapon of Wahl with a look of half-surprise, half-panic on her face.

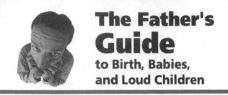
Chapter Three

Tyler, in the classic head-down position of ignorant haircut bliss, was totally unaware that the back of his head now featured a matching pair of to-the-skin stripes extending a couple inches straight up from the bottom of his hairline. It was as if someone had rammed a high-revving power mower head-on into a batch of tall weeds, leaving a mower-wide notch in the middle of the weed bed.

For some reason, emergency hair repair was not a featured segment of the Wahl video.

Trying her best to not alert Tyler or laugh out loud, Karen subtly communicated the point of not saying anything to hurt his feelings as she attempted to smooth out, fill in and otherwise cover the not-so-slight imperfection.

Thanks to the feigned attempts at nonchalance, much laughter-halting lip-biting and no mirrors in the kitchen, Tyler's first home haircut was completed with the illusion of success.

Until Hayley promptly burst on the scene with an exclamation of little girl honesty and loudly yelled, "Mom, how come you cut a big 'M' in the back of his head when his name starts with 'T'?"

Good question, but it could have been worse. It could have been a Beatles' haircut.

Behind Schedule As Scheduled

One of the first things discovered by new parents is that once children are involved, everything not only takes much longer than planned, it takes much longer than you could imagine.

Our New Year's resolution for the past seven New Year's has been to simply to be on time, preferably more than once, although once would be a nice start.

It's also highly unlikely.

As near as we can figure out, we next expect to be on time for anything in the year 2017, at which time our undoers of child-proof locks will be 18, 21 and 23, respectively, and hopefully able to load the minivan.

Until then, don't count on us for dinner, unless it's for breakfast.

Our road to wherever is always paved with the proverbial good intentions, but we have a hard time finding the entrance ramp.

Keeping Up Appearances

Excursions are pre-planned, planned, checked and double-checked, but you can count on death, taxes and us being two hours late.

This is fine if you're running a major airline, but a bit trying for those whose daily lives revolve around routine or some other alien concept.

Part of the problem, of course, is the logistical nightmare of packing. We do not visit people, we descend upon them, a five-person invasion force armed with portable cribs, booster chairs, walkers and the wardrobe of a touring musical. Mismatched suitcases bulge with contingencies for every forecast – warm, cold, wet or dry. Long pants, short pants, snow pants, no pants, sweaters and T-shirts fight for space along with the obligatory must-be-seen-in outfits that so-and-so sent for Arbor Day. The urp factor demands that two of everything be carried.

Menu planning (see urp factor above) for the highchair set also requires a hefty payload. As such, no urban hillbilly roadshow would be complete without a couple of weak-bottomed paper grocery bags containing dozens of jars of assorted fruits and vegetables, each smashed, blended and pureed beyond recognition or taste. Accompanying utensils such as miniature spoons, covered cups, plastic plates and bibs are tossed into a separate bag, to be forgotten later on the kitchen counter.

This gets us to the door.

Loading the van is an exact science based on mathematics where cubic feet divided by the number of items minus "Do we really need this?" equals the amount of stuff carried back into the house.

Actually locking the front door results in a phenomenon that cannot be explained by science or The Learning Channel. For some reason, the turning of the key and clicking of the lock activates all prunes eaten over the last four weeks by everyone under the age of seven. Clean diapers are without fail stashed in whatever suitcase is buried on the bottom of the van. As they say at Cape Canaveral, this delays the launch.

Re-opening the front door triggers an avalanche of phone calls, usually from a telemarketer asking to speak to "the denture wearer of the house," or from a panicking relative who figures the next time they see our van-loaded entourage will be on the side of a milk carton.

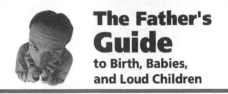

Chapter Three

This was the case when we opted for a visit to my parents' house in northern Wisconsin, although a month-long trip up the Amazon would have been easier.

Our hoped-for time of departure was daylight.

With an early morning start on our 700 trips to the van and the obligatory finishing of several dozen last-minute things that each takes 20 minutes, we were close to being on schedule as dusk approached when the phone rang somewhere around the umpteenth locking of the front door.

After two siding salesmen, a carpet-cleaning offer and three wrong numbers, this call had the distinctive ring of my mother.

Despite our track record, she seemed somewhat surprised that we were still home to answer the phone, especially since the potatoes we were supposed to be eating would done in 10 minutes in an oven 240 miles away.

No problem.

As we'll be saying for the next 15 years or so, "We'll get there when we get there."

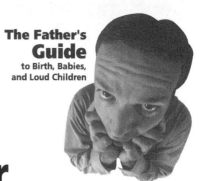

Chapter Four

Lines Of Communication

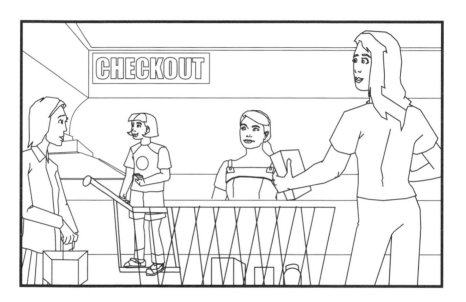

Hurdling the Language Barrier

One of the highlights of infancy is the first sound other than crying that escapes from the baby. Usually it's some sort of cooing sound, a soft, gentle, reassuring noise of contentment that is unmatched in heart-warming capability.

As babies discover that their tongue can be used for more than producing copious amounts of slobber, the cooing sound changes from a solid, gentle monotone to a mixture of vowel sounds running up and down the musical scale, much like the conversational ability of the last guy to leave the frat party.

In most instances, the first consonant to leap into the conversational picture is the "D" sound, a soft, whisper-like "dah" that most men immediately take as "SHE SAID, DAD!!! SHE DID!!! SHE SAID DAD."

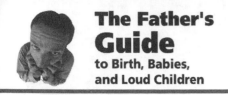
Chapter Four

Even though this is not the case, it still hacks off the new mom who has done 99 percent of the work up to this point.

At some point, when lip control improves a little bit, the first "M" sound will be followed by the word, mom. In fact, it often becomes a non-stop running mom, mom, mom, mom, mom for hours on end.

Eventually the "M" sound also will be applied to dad, usually at the beginning of the word "money," as in, "Dad, I need money ... lots and lots of money."

Every child also goes through the "no" phase in which every question, statement or sentence is answered with a polite, but firmly unshakable no. This phase miraculously passes right before your patience is about to expire for good.

The ultimate parental crusher, which will eventually spout forth, is the first time that your pride and joy, your adorable little boy or girl, looks right at you and says, "I hate you," in his or her most petulant tone. Trust me on this one, it will happen, but it will still catch you totally off balance. Minutes later they may turn to the family dog, a brother or a sister and also tell them, "I hate you."

In most instances, the child has no concept of what he or she actually said, but many a psychiatrist has made the payment on the Porsche from a parent whose fragile psyche was shattered by the first, "I hate you."

Eventually, kids will grow to know what they're saying and blurt out an equally surprising, unconditional, "I love you."

That's what keeps you going.

Repeat After Me

As soon as your children learn to talk, there will be no such thing as a family secret. In short order, the whole world will know everything about any subject discussed within the four walls of your house or anywhere else where your children can hear the conversation. And, there will be no topic off limits, such as when dad needs new underwear.

After a couple years of utterly charming and relatively innocent toddler chatter, Hayley in one overnight move became a non-stop

Lines Of Communication

walking, talking echo machine; a three-foot tall human tape recorder of unerring accuracy with a playback button timed for ultimate embarrassment.

The locker-room axiom of "What you hear here stays here when you leave here," does not apply to those who wear the uniforms of Baby B'Gosh.

Each bit of juicy gossip, catty criticism or off-color remark previously uttered in the complete confidence of your own cluttered kitchen now runs the risk of being repeated at full volume in a public place.

Admittedly, this concept is nothing new. In fact, the simple realization of this children-to-parents embarrassment potential kept Art Linkletter atop the world of black-and-white TV for years.

As a result, however, veteran parents have long since learned to talk in code, spelling out entire paragraphs punctuated with the rolling eyes, discrete head jerks and subtle hand gestures of a spastic, stressed-out mime ... J-O-C-K-I-T-C-H, twitch, twitch, twitch.

Rudimentary foreign language skills, such as pidgin-Spanish, also are extremely useful. For example, widening the eyes to the size of pie tins and puffing your cheeks like trumpeter Dizzy Gillespie in breathless search of a high note, along with the simple Spanish word, "baño" is child-proof code for "I need to use the bathroom NOW without an audience, you hold the kids."

Gracias.

As with everything else, some of these tricks are learned only by example. In the lexicon of parenting, this also is known as learning the hard way.

With a background that includes, but is not limited to, military service, sports writing, rugby and barroom singer-songwriter, it is not surprising that I at least have working knowledge of what my grandmother politely referred to as "salty language."

Nevertheless, it was still quite a surprise the first time Hayley surveyed the daily post-hurricane look of our living room, calmly put both hands on hips and loudly proclaimed in her best drill-instructor voice, "Goldarn mess."

Except she didn't say that, exactly. Nope. It was the full-fledged, truck-stop, bang-your-knuckles-when-the-wrench-slips version of "goldarn."

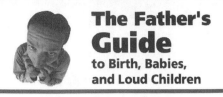

Chapter Four

After a brief moment of wondering about the hereditary impact of old George Carlin albums, I realized that this was not a phrase picked up from me, at least not in that context. A fumble during a televised Packers game, yes, but a household mess, no. My wife will readily, if unfortunately, attest to the fact that when it comes to laundry piles (and four million other things) that I easily assume the role of Mr. Oblivious.

As such, the finger of guilt in this instance pointed directly at the only other adult in our house. The rarity of this not only made the situation understandable, but from my point of view, it was downright hilarious, although not to be encouraged.

Since then, golly, gee, shucks, shoot, darn, dangit have reestablished themselves in our daily vocabulary. Only a strand of pearls and a tube of Brylcream stand between us and the Cleavers.

The parroting ability of toddlers is not limited to the occasional slip of barracks-type language. Seemingly innocent and innocuous phrases are stored away for later use like an out-of-context TV talkshow soundbite (speaking of which, where is Art Linkletter when you really need him?)

Visitors to the front door are loudly and enthusiastically greeted with, "I have BMs" or "Hi, the dog threw up." Complete strangers now are privy to the family's best-kept secrets.

To give mom (not mine, Hayley's, Tyler's and Colin's) a well-deserved, much-needed ... I-M-G-O-I-N-G-C-R-A-Z-Y, twitch, twitch ... break, we headed out for a stroller-loaded afternoon of lunch and shopping.

As we cleaned up the remnants of an appetizing smorgasbord that included smashed prunes, two french fries, some smeared applesauce and three bites of hot dog, the waitress politely asked Hayley about her afternoon plans.

Without hesitation she proudly and clearly answered with her best just-turned-2 enunciation, "We going shopping. Papa needs new underwear. It has holes in it."

The waitress thought it was, well, pretty goldarn funny.

Workout At The Why

With each of our children, we also went through a demanding daily exercise routine known as the workout at the why.

From early morning's first crib-side cry of, "I'm awake," to the final reassuring good-night reply of, "Do I have to come in there?" every in-between waking moment was spent in a non-stop verbal sparring session with mom and dad bobbing and weaving through the continuous questioning barrage of why, why, why and more why.

When Hayley zeroed in on her third birthday, no person, place, or thing was an off-limits topic, no matter how embarrassing from an adult point of view. Nothing was left to chance, everything was questioned. Living in our house was like hosting an eternal version of Jeopardy. The categories were endless and total strangers were politely invited to play along. Unfortunates trapped behind us in the checkout line at the supermarket invariably became participants, usually in the "Wardrobe" category. Unsuspecting daydreamers were unceremoniously jerked from their non-paying perusal of *People* magazine by our cart-confined version of Alex Trabek.

"Why are you wearing black shoes?"

"I beg your pardon?" someone, anyone, was forced to answer as they noticed Hayley pointing at their feet.

"Why are you wearing black shoes?

"Oh, because I like to."

"Do they match your black car?"

"My car is white."

"Is your dog white, too?"

"What? Oh no, we don't have a dog."

"If you had a white dog, would he chew on your black shoes?"

At that point, even the most polite person usually sought refuge behind the nearest trashy tabloid paper, suddenly enthralled by that week's celebrity divorces. Others nonchalantly scanned the remaining checkout aisles, eventually choosing to stand in an even longer, slower-

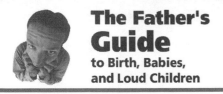

Chapter Four

moving line rather than face another round of totally disjointed questions. Some simply abandoned their fully-laden carts, forfeiting their chance at Final Jeopardy.

Undaunted, the questioning simply shifted back to mom or dad.

"Why that lady was wearing black shoes?"

Two aisles away, the black-shoed woman in the slow-moving line smirked in question-free bliss.

Actually attempting to answer a why question usually makes it worse. One misstep and you are suddenly up to your ears in conversational quicksand.

During one festive holiday season, I was relying on a compact disc of Christmas music to help entertain Hayley and Tyler, who, at the time was still thankfully in the pre-why stage.

Anyway, a wonderful children's choir was interrupted in mid rump-a-bump-bum by Hayley, who wanted to know why the little drummer boy was playing his drum.

At the risk of religious inaccuracy, my off-hand answer had something to do with the fact that the little drummer boy didn't have any money and, as such, was offering his music as a special gift.

This seemingly innocuous answer triggered an avalanche of loud, deep sobs as Hayley emotionally asked, "Why the little drummer boy doesn't have any money?"

Each successive answer was more in-depth and detailed than the last, but failed to stem the tide of tears.

By the time calm had been restored, my lengthy and borderline blasphemous question-by-question explanation of the little drummer boy's financial plight was sort of that he didn't have any money, but his parent's did, but they were at work and he couldn't get a hold of them on his cell phone and he didn't have a cash card for the ATM, but he was carrying his drum to work because his band had a party gig and they were going to play "Happy Birthday" for a certain newborn baby boy.

That's why.

The Antics Of Semantics

"What we have here is a failure to communicate."

Hollywood made the line famous, but it was no doubt inspired by a sit-down, hash-it-out, heart-to-heart, toddler-to-parent chat in which the adult had exactly no clue as to what on earth was being discussed.

And, no amount of animated clue-giving can guide a slow-to-catch-on adult through the Mixmaster sentence structure of a two-year-old's vocabulary. Verbs, nouns and all other grammatical terms are infinitely interchangeable, while tense refers only to the frustration level of the non-understanding parent.

As soon as she could talk, Hayley's rapidly expanding vocabulary often was used to provide up-to-the-minute reports on the status of her younger brothers.

While she was still mastering the finer points of tattling, she joined an adults-only conversation to point out that Tyler had "a grobber."

Grobber?

"Uh, huh. Him got a grobber," she repeated, patiently waiting for my response.

Like a computerized dictionary, my mind sorted through option after option, "Grabber? Grumbler?"

"Uh, huh. Him got a grobber. By his nose."

One quick glance at Tyler solved the linguistic mystery. I'm still not sure where she'd originally picked up the intended word, but it was clear she meant to point out that her younger brother was, indeed, the proud possessor of a world-class booger.

Or in this instance, "grobber," and "Thank you, Hayley, for pointing that out."

Despite the occasional phonetic mix-up, Hayley usually managed to eventually get her point across. Prior to actual conversation ability, Tyler tended to rely on a mixture of points, grunts and screeches to discuss anything other than "ball," the one word he consistently nailed on a daily basis.

Tyler, would you like some cantaloupe?

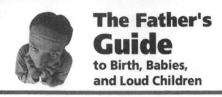
Chapter Four

"Ball."

Tyler, would you like an apple?

"Ball."

Tyler, don't pull on the dog's head.

"Ball."

And so on and so on and so on.

Geographic differences also come into conversational play, such as the similar difference between bubbler and drinking fountain or, in this instance, soda and pop.

To keep conversational air as clear as possible, we've tried to steer some of our children's grammatical choices away from the more blatantly embarrassing phrases. Take flatulence, for example. (Now there's a sentence you don't type everyday). We are talking here, of course, about the shyly innocent toddler version of passing gas, not the four-octave, bean-fueled, Blazing Saddles campfire chorus.

When that occurs, we have so far gotten away with having them politely saying in their cutest, I-can-get-away-with-it, I'm-a-little-kid-voice, "I popped, excuse me."

"I popped." Simple and polite. No muss, no fuss, no locker room jokes.

During one visit to my parents' house, Hayley was busy "playing dishes," plying her dolls with imaginary delights from a variety of empty cups and plates. When my dad walked into the living room, cola in hand, and spotted Hayley's empty glass, he politely offered, "Hayley, would you like some pop in that glass?"

The look of astonishment on Hayley's face as she mulled over that offer clearly indicated that she thought that would be quite a trick, possibly worthy of Lettermen and infinitely more entertaining than the old, "Pull my finger," routine.

"Pop? In my cup?" followed by as much crinkling as a button nose can muster, all the while looking for an answer from yours truly, whose face was buried three feet into a laughter-hiding pillow. Unfortunately, I couldn't stick around to resolve the situation. Tyler had a grobber that needed attention.

The Land Of Loud

In moving from one elementary school generation to the next, the traditional three Rs of readin', 'riting and 'rithmetic have been replaced by one L.

Loud.

Not specific loud, just loud in general.

From sunup to sundown, our entire house vibrates from the sonic output of three active children. Anything and everything is done at the auditory level of a heavy metal concert.

It doesn't matter who is up the earliest, although that is usually reserved for Tyler, whose self-proclaimed official job is to be the first one up.

On his own, he sneaks out of his room and climbs into a kid-battered recliner simply known as "the green chair." He then curls up and waits in surprisingly quiet solitude for the pitter-patter of a second set of little feet.

Although he is quiet on the outside, the noise pressure apparently is building up inside, ready to be released in a geyser of house-waking sound at the first appearance of either Hayley or Colin.

"GOOD MORNING, HAYLEY!!" shouted with all the subtlety of Ozzie Osbourne taking the stage. His early morning enthusiasm usually is tempered by an exaggerated stage-whisper admonishment from the adult bedroom.

"Tyler!! Shhhhhh!!! Whisper, please. Other people are sleeping."

His barely heard reply of, "OK," is, of course, followed by, "GOOD MORNING, COLIN!!"

From a vocal standpoint, our day, and that of most of the surrounding neighborhood, is underway and it only gets louder.

By some miracle, the three of them actually manage to eat breakfast, although their mouths are never actually closed. In an effort to be heard above the others, they approach conversation under the theory of Tijuana taxi drivers where the loudest horn has the right of way. Our breakfast table is a busy intersection. Adults do not read the morning paper, they hide under it. Why read the comic strips when you live them?

With Hayley and Tyler off on the school bus, the noise level drops considerably for a brief period of time as Colin's 3-year-old noisemaking ability is pretty much limited to knocking things over and falling down, although his vocabulary and lung power are simultaneously expanding.

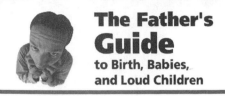

Chapter Four

The end of relative quiet coincides with the return of Tyler's school bus, his mouth opening in synchronization with the folding bus door.

"HEY, DAD," he hollers, as if I were standing in another zip code. "WANT TO SEE WHAT A BOY TAUGHT ME ON THE BUS?"

Being an involved parent, I, of course, say sure, as if I have a choice.

Tyler then proceeds to put his wrists together, puff out his cheeks, put his mouth in the combined palms of his hands and blow as hard as he can, instantly producing a 45-second burst of world-class simulated flatulence.

I must admit that, for a beginner, he was awfully good.

By the end of the afternoon, he had passed on his newly acquired skill to Colin, whose efforts, although sincere, produced more slobber than sound.

Because Hayley is still in school in the afternoons, Tyler occasionally invites another kindergarten boy over to play. The activity of choice appears to involve nothing more than running aimlessly around the front yard yelling nonsensical syllables at the top of their lungs, stopping occasionally to pick up a "whapping" stick.

In other words, much like a training class for corporate managers.

When afternoon Bus No. 2 arrives with Hayley, the "how was your day?" process repeats itself, except she has to yell loud enough to be heard over the shouts of her brothers.

The limited time between school and dinner is spent in a variety of activities, the only requirement being that they are loud.

Sometimes it involves musical instruments, sometimes a fleet of relative-given toy trucks, each requiring approximately 37 AA batteries to operate the real-sounding sirens and horns.

Usually, however, it is simply a loud, top-of-the-lung argument over who had which toy first. When properly motivated, Colin can cry louder than either Hayley or Tyler can yell.

Based on noise alone, it is not surprising that our children like to sing, particularly in the so-called quiet time before bed. In an effort to promote family harmony, I introduced them to a long-ago favorite from my own school bus-riding days.

"Greasy, grimy pieces of gopher guts ..."

Judging by the fall-off-the-bed response of Hayley, Tyler and Colin, it is still a showstopper. And remember, you don't have to be good if you're loud.

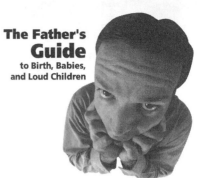

Chapter Five

Health & Nutrition

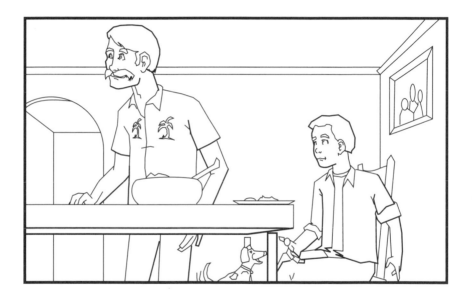

Feeding Frenzy

The entire spectrum of children's eating habits can be boiled down into two simple categories: Good Eaters and Picky Eaters. Good Eaters, as the name implies, will willingly sample almost anything placed in front of them regardless of color, texture or ethnic origin. Picky Eaters, on the other hand, usually exist for most of their pre-teen years on one or two staple items such as cereal or peanut butter, deflecting all other nutritional obligations with a straightforward, "I don't like that."

Few people on earth are as smug as parents whose children fall into the Good Eaters category. But eating habits, like everything else associated with parenting, have a way of evening themselves out.

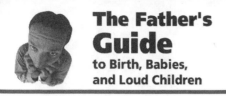
Chapter Five

In our house, after years of good-eating, table top harmony, we suddenly found ourselves locked in nightly tussles over each and every dinner plate. In the terminology of high chair battlefields, we had met the enemy and it was rice.

After almost always eating anything plopped in front of them, as well as the occasional dust-based floor appetizer, our children suddenly became culinary connoisseurs, jointly turning up their noses at a wide range of foods that previously were scarfed down by the ton.

Especially rice, of any kind, and accompanying beans, whether they be red, black or pinto.

Since spoons first became their plastic-handled weapons of choice, our kids had without discrimination attacked heaping helpings of everything from artichokes to zucchini.

No sauce was too saucy and few spices too spicy as they spilled, splattered and sprayed their way through each of the basic food groups. Their willingness to sample anything at any time was a source of pride as we smugly watched other parents tackle the dreaded one-track appetite of children who would eat nothing but macaroni and cheese, peanut butter and jelly or oatmeal.

Hayley, Tyler and Colin, on the other hand, were like a three-person United Nations delegation when it came to the dinner table.

Italian pastas of any shape and size were devoured by the plateful, accompanied by the rallying cry of, "Holy Moly ravioli." Mountains of Chinese food disappeared pea pod by pea pod. Fiesta-sized platters of tacos, enchiladas and burritos were consumed on weekly runs for the border.

After a romp through the international buffet, good ol' American cuisine such as hamburgers, hot dogs, soup and sandwiches were an easily accomplished walk on the mild side. Breakfast, lunch and dinner were matter-of-factly handled without argument and, surprisingly, often without dessert.

Considering that our children rarely had seen dad without a candy bar, brownie, cookie, doughnut or other large chunk of solidified sugar, dessert-free anything in our house was almost beyond belief.

(My wife takes a much more scientific approach to the dessert tray. While recently perusing the point-of-purchase candy rack at the grocery store checkout line, she made the startling discovery that a bag of

Health & Nutrition

M&M's has less sugar than certain brands of yogurt. She mathematically concluded, of course, that M&M's were definitely better for a person than was yogurt. We are now working on the Snickers bar versus lettuce salad comparison.)

But, on the main-course front, rice and beans, whether they be red, black or pinto, were a quick and easy, last-minute answer to "what's for dinner?"

In one 24-hour span, however, the answer changed.

Suddenly, rice and the aforementioned rainbow coalition of beans were off-limits, persona non grata on the high chair tray. Formerly active spoons sat stubbornly idle as if manned by union eaters on strike.

As a result, I found myself passing on the generation-to-generation threat, "You're not getting out of that chair until you're done eating."

This, of course, is a lesson carried over from my own childhood when I could handle rice, but not pork chops. The only difference was that I was told I would sit there until the "pork chops were gone," not until "I was done eating."

Although the difference in phrasing may have been a fine distinction of Bill Clintonesque proportions, to me it meant early parole for the prisoner of pork chops.

Left alone and unsupervised at the formica-topped kitchen table, I methodically cut the offending pork chop into half-inch squares and promptly stuffed the pieces down the nearest hollow chrome table leg.

When the authoritative voice from the other room again asked if the pork chop was gone, I truthfully, if somewhat Presidentially, answered, "Yes."

My indiscretion went undiscovered for the better part of a decade until the purchase of a new kitchen table. When my dad removed the legs from the old table, a few dozen or so chunks of petrified something or other bounced across the kitchen floor. Only one person on the face of the earth recognized them as the long-buried evidence of uneaten pork chops.

Now, more than three decades later, the ghost of pork chops past once again had reared its ugly head.

Ironically, one of Karen's specialties is a family recipe for pork chops and rice. The kids and I have had some long, long meals.

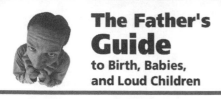
Chapter Five

Dog Day Afternoon

When it comes to life, liberty and the pursuit of hot dogs, it is never too early to become an activist.

At the politically correct age of 2 1/2, Tyler decided to fix what he perceived to be one of the great fast food injustices of the Midwest.

After finally exhausting my supply of excuses, Tuesdays became dad and Tyler day at swim class. After a half-hour of scoops, kicks, bubbles, jumps, torpedoes and "Little pig, little pig, let me in," we mini-vanned our way to our weekly guys-only lunch, which had better, as I discovered, include a hot dog, or else.

If we hustled through the post-swim class routine without losing a sock, the car keys or my patience, grabbing a hot dog was a metaphor-mixing piece of cake. Less than two mouth-watering minutes away from the YMCA was a local deli that housed an Oscar Mayer grilling station, a glass-encased treasure trove filled to the steamy seams with rack after rack of kid-attracting hot dogs.

With the prospect of a hot dog literally just around the corner, post-swim class appetites were whetted at the top of our lungs with an entire Hit Parade of sing-along appetizers.

"I wish I were an Oscar Mayer wiener ... "

"Hot dogs, Armour hot dogs, what kind of kids eat Armour hot dogs ... "

"Hot diggity, dog diggity, boom, what you do to me, boom, what you do to me..."

By the time we reached the deli parking lot, Tyler had sung himself into a complete pre-hot dog frenzy.

One quick sweep through the store and we were set. Hot dog, mustard, ketchup, potato chips, milk, cookie. The perfect guy lunch. Not a salad bar in sight. Talk with your mouth full. Wipe your hands on your pants. And, most importantly, no older, domineering cookie-grabbing sister around with whom he was forced to share.

After one grueling swim class, we offset the fact that we were five minutes later than our usual five minutes late by staying for an extra 15 minutes of pool time. Little did I know the price of the so-called free swim.

Health & Nutrition

We arrived at the deli just as the hot dog-consuming construction crews were leaving. As Tyler zoomed around the corner of the counter, his sprint for the promised land was halted in mid Stride-Rite stride.

The grilling station was empty!!

Tyler's expression was that of the dumbfounded Geraldo Rivera when he discovered that Al Capone's vault was, indeed, empty.

Recognizing the misty eyes and quivering lower lip as the warning signals of a complete toddler meltdown, I immediately switched to the cheer up, it'll be all right mode with the guarantee that we would find another hot dog.

Except we couldn't.

We drove from one prospective hot dog outlet to the next with no luck. From convenience store to convenience store, mini-mart to gas station through one fast food drive-through after another, the answer, as unfathomable as it seemed, was the same. No hot dogs.

With the gas gauge and the patience meter both on empty, we finally settled on a McDonald's drive through. When the almost-decipherable speaker voice asked for our order, Tyler, of course, screamed for a hot dog.

Several minutes of argument ensued between the static-crackling speaker and a stubborn pint-sized supporter of hot dog rights. All the while the guy in the car behind us pounded on his steering wheel, silently mouthing what I'm guessing were I'm-in-a-hurry obscenities.

We finally settled on a small order of Chicken McNuggets, which remained uneaten under the van seat for several months.

A couple weeks later, Tyler got into a lengthy locker room conversation with a nice older gentleman about the afternoon plans, which Tyler said included lunch with dad.

When the man mistakenly mentioned the golden arches, Tyler, in the voice of the truly indignant, immediately informed him that he was going to write a letter to McDonald's. That was news to me.

Trying to keep a straight face, the guy asked Tyler what the letter was going to say. It was short, sweet and to the point.

"Dear McDonald's, I think you should have hot dogs for kids. Tyler."

With several years of swimming classes still ahead of us, I couldn't agree more.

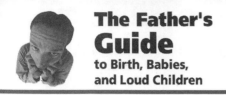

Chapter Five

School Spirit Is Contagious

An entire nation of educational consultants is correct about the immediate effect of pre-school attendance on first-time students.

Within 24 hours of first setting foot in a classroom, results are noticeable.

Welcome to class, here's your germs. 19,457 different kinds of them. Please take them home and give them to your parents. The tissue paper industry thanks you.

Like most parents who had not slept in slightly more than three years, any concerns about enrolling our Hayley in pre-school were balanced by prospects of the first parental afternoon nap since 1994. In addition to the purely educational aspects of such a move, the mere thought of a chatter-free afternoon of relaxation was, admittedly, somewhat of a factor in the final decision.

After a lengthy interview process ("No, that was some other Gray clan that burned the castle in 1412"), our application and checking account were approved.

(At the same time we were filling out Hayley's pre-school application, I was in the midst of a space-making, throw-the-old-stuff-away day. In a drawer that should have been labeled, "Do I need this junk?" I came across the receipt from my first semester at one of the state university schools from which I eventually graduated without honor. The cost of that entire 16 1/2-credit semester at what is known worldwide as the Harvard of Cheeseland was roughly one-half that of the three-day-a-week semester of pre-school singalongs and finger painting.)

Anyway, with financial reality firmly, if somewhat shockingly, established, our previously homebound little girl was off on the path to eventual higher education.

At the end of the first day of class, we, along with 47 other minivan-driving parents, eagerly awaited the initial report.

"Hayley, how was your first day of school?"

"I didn't listen and one boy sneezed."

Health & Nutrition

From the standpoint of the proverbial student-teacher relationship, Day One with our pint-sized Miss Stubborn apparently could have gone better, but for those invested in the pharmaceutical industry, it was, as they say, a red-letter day on Wall Street.

Less than one day after Hayley's introduction to preschool, everyone of voting age in our house had learned the caught-it-from-the-kids ABCs.

A is for antihistamine because your nose is stuffed up,

B is for Benadryl, which you drink by the cup,

C is for Cold-Eeze to make your sneeze quit,

D is for decongestant because you feel like . . . shoot me and put me out of my misery.

And, by adult standards, preschool or grade school generated colds are much more determined than the grown-up, take-a-pill, feel-better-in-the-morning variety.

Childhood colds make an adult nose run like a marathon trainee. Plumbers charge two zillion dollars an hour to stop similar drips. Despite advertising claims to the contrary, even the softest tissue is the same grit used in wood finishing. As your head is about to explode, you realize why George Carlin once did a bit called "Snot, the original rubber cement."

It takes a special person to put a positive spin on such medical misery. Someone like former cowboy singer, now mystery novelist, Richard "Kinky" Friedman.

In his current persona as a cigar-smoking fictional gumshoe, the Kinkster is the hippest of the hip, shoot from the lip of literary crime solvers, relying on puns and one liners instead of fisticuffs. His novels, starring himself, include such staples of our bookshelf as *The Love Song of J. Edgar Hoover* and *God Bless John Wayne*.

Before becoming a black-clad darling of the bookstore set, however, Kinky Friedman fronted one of the most bizarre musical outfits in the history of country music. As such, his albums still occupy a special place in my alphabetized, pre-CD collection.

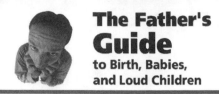
Chapter Five

With our household knee-deep in used Kleenex, I trotted out one of the old Kinky Friedman standards, "Ol' Ben Lucas," to the delight of the kids.

On the original recording, the song is performed with a children's choir, accompanied by a plink, plink, plinking toy piano like that played by Schroeder in the Peanuts cartoons.

Within minutes, the kids were joining in at the top of their lungs.

"Ol' Ben Lucas, had a lot of mucus, comin' right out of his nose . . ."

Singalong time at school probably will never be the same. I figure it's a fair trade for the germs.

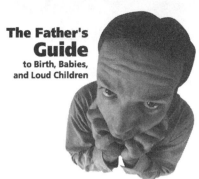

Chapter Six

They Must Get It From Their Mother

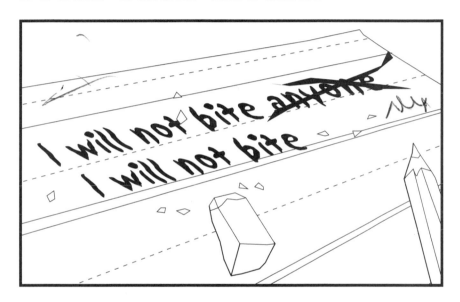

The Write, Write, Write Stuff

Less than a month into the unexplored territory of first grade, it appeared that our daughter, Hayley, was a chip off the old writer's block.

Much like her father, except, of course for the bad haircut and worse wardrobe, she had taken the first literary steps down the path toward limited earning power.

During one writing exercise, she was the picture of concentration, pen curled tightly in hand, tongue tip protruding from the corner of her mouth, squinted eyes focusing on the wide-lined paper as she carefully and methodically shaped each letter under my watchful editorial eye.

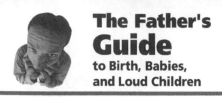
Chapter Six

I will not spit.

I will not spit.

I will not spit.

And so on and so on down to the 25th and final line of the page.

It may not have been Beatrix Potter, but it did get the message across that siblings, neighbor children and the family dog were not appropriate targets.

It also took me on a Ked-wearing, Schwinn-riding trip down memory lane to my own grade school days when the first four gazillion written words of my life began with the phrase "I will not," followed by a line-by-line promise not to repeat whatever it was I had done.

My hand actually cramped as the faces of justice flashed through my memory – Mrs. Bowen, Mrs. Smith, Miss Worth, Miss Reed, Mrs. Endresen – a grade-by-grade parade of ruler-wielding editorial authority. In serving my sentences of sentences, I filled dozens of Indian Chief writing tablets from front to back with thousands of lines of I will not something-or-other.

I will not push. I will not talk back. I will not fight. I will not talk back. I will not use my Bic pen to shoot spitwads. I will not talk back. I will not read Mad magazine in class. I will not talk back. Some lessons took longer than others to sink in.

Later newsroom pressure would pale in comparison to maintaining journalistic composure in front of an entire snickering class as my trademark "I will nots" filled the blackboard.

If I had been particularly obnoxious, as to which most childhood friends would attest was often the case, I would get to erase all of my chalk-based handiwork and start over, an early, but effective, example of self-editing.

They Must Get It From Their Mother

At the end of the school day, parole was gained by cleaning all the erasers, maniacally clapping them together to create huge, swirling yellow clouds of chalk dust, which were later suspected as a primary cause of acid rain.

In family annals, two other early writing attempts stand out.

The first was when my mom came off the front porch to find me admiring a carefully crafted four-letter effort.

Although I am a bit fuzzy on the actual details, I apparently had been contentedly drawing with a piece of sandstone on the sidewalk when an older boy came by and whispered letter by letter what I should write.

Once I got past "F", the rest was easy. It was the first, but certainly not the last, thing I wrote of which my mother disapproved. To this day I also have a well-earned wariness of assignment editors.

My second faux pas occurred when the Cub Scout manual did not specifically prohibit out-and-out forgery. In my haste to obtain the much-sought-after Wolf Badge, I went through each of the book's required tasks and filled in the signature blank.

I may not have been much of a knot-tyer, but I could write my mom's name.

Of course, since it was written in the large, loopy scrawl of a third-grader, the ruse was quickly discovered. My large, loopy scrawl did improve, however, after several hundred lines of "I will not sign my mother's name."

I am proud to report that Hayley's penmanship efforts are continuing in hereditary fashion. I recently found her seated at the kitchen table working on a line-by-line assignment given by my wife.

I will not bite anyone.

I will not bite anyone.

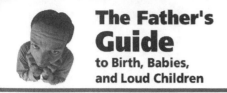
Chapter Six

This proved to be not only a bit wordy, but a tad long in first-grade writing style for the width of the paper. Displaying great initiative, Hayley simply went back to the original sentence, crossed out the word anyone and moved the period.

The new sentence now read, "I will not bite." I thought it was well edited.

To Push Or Not To Push

When William Shakespeare penned the phrase, "All the world's a stage," I'm not sure if he meant to include the local Walgreens.

But, that's exactly where Tyler turned in one of his best dramatic performances to date. Right there in aisle 8c amidst the cavity-fighting ambiance of dental care products.

The production started as a short jaunt to what was formerly known as the corner drug store, which, of course, is now a Walgreens that dots every corner of America.

Because Tyler's early goal in life is to become an honors graduate from the diesel truck driving school, he is enamored and wildly enthusiastic about anything with wheels. As such, his first request at every retail outlet was to push the shopping cart. For whatever reason, be it his lack of steering ability, the possibility that his little brother might topple out, aisles crowded with senior citizens, or simply the parental trump card of, "Because I said so," Karen denied his request.

Although normally easy-going and pleasant, Tyler, like every kindergartner, has his moments. This was one of them. He responded to the denial by throwing what my late grandmother referred to as a "conniption fit," but which most people basically call a tantrum. But this was no run-of-the mill temper display with such amateurish effects as crying, foot-stomping or holding of breath.

They Must Get It From Their Mother

This was improvisational theater at its finest, a gripping conflict between the immovable pint-sized object and the irresistible parental force.

After being told that he couldn't push the cart, Tyler weaseled his way between Karen and the handle under the theory that assisted pushing is better than no pushing at all. The prospect of walking awkwardly through the entire store with 6-inch steps held surprisingly little appeal for Karen, so she politely asked him to relinquish his co-pilot's role.

In the family game of one-upmanship, Tyler countered by suddenly dropping to the floor, lying motionless on his side amongst the Crest and Colgate, Oral-B and Reach. After the usual array of stage-whispered threats, Karen decided the best option was to ignore him and roll forward.

Hayley, as the big sister, took her role as the family whistle-blower quite seriously, keeping an on eye on Tyler with a running verbal update easily heard by everyone in the store.

"He's still lying there."

"He hasn't moved."

"Tyler, you're acting like such a kid."

When Karen started to regain the upper hand, Tyler switched to the old "oblivious walk in the other direction" tactic. As would every safety-minded parent, Karen quickly corralled him with the stipulation that he keep one hand on the cart at all times.

In a brilliant, double-meaning display of dramatic resistance, Tyler did, indeed, keep one hand on the cart, while the entire rest of his body went completely limp. As gravity took over, Tyler slowly slumped to his knees, his one mandatory hand the lone lifeline to the Walgreens shopping cart.

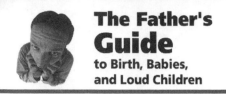

Chapter Six

Rather than continue the argument, Karen slowly inched the cart, and Tyler, forward. Like a wounded cowboy hanging on to the buckboard, Tyler dragged alongside, the knees of his school pants leaving two clearly marked trails on the dusty tile floor.

As Karen's patience neared its end, Tyler's survival instincts took over and, as if blessed by a faith healer, he miraculously regained his feet, bringing down the curtain on another family production.

But that was just the opening act. He now focuses his efforts on the big family grocery shopping trips where the carts are piled to the ceiling with enough food for a small country or our family of five. To push or not to push, that is the question.

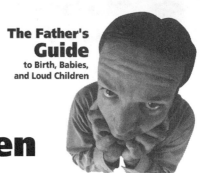

Chapter Seven

He Learned It From His Father

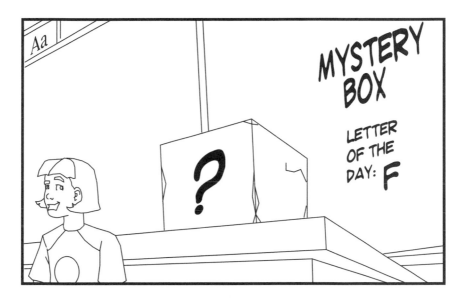

Licensed Immaturity

When it comes to fatherly legacy, lunacy is in the eye of the beholder.

Depending upon your viewpoint, the time-honored tradition of stuff passing on from fathers to their children is either really neat or just plain stupid.

The equation is remarkably simple. Male viewpoint = really neat. Female viewpoint = just plain stupid.

For example, if, after watching a boy-caused neighborhood disaster that involved loud noises, descriptions of bodily functions or petroleum products, a guy will beam with absolute pride as he overhears another guy say, "He learned that from his father."

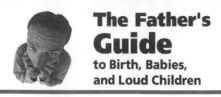
Chapter Seven

If a female witnesses the exact same scene, she is apt to utter the exact same, "He learned that from his father," proclaimed with all the disgust, embarrassment and judgment-passing a human voice can contain.

The simple fact is that in some aspects of life the gender gap is as wide as the Grand Canyon and as evenly divided as a junior high dance.

To the best of my recollection, in every single classroom in which I was ever seated, whether it was row-by-row, alphabetical or tallest in the back, I cannot remember one single female who stuffed her hand into her armpit to create world-class simulated flatulence. Not even the most tommish of tomboys chose to participate in this particular endeavor. Nope, this boys-think-funny, girls-think-classless act was solely the domain of a male, usually four or five of them, flailing away in the back of a classroom like an evolutionary experiment gone sadly awry.

In the eyes of the opposite sex, that image has come back to haunt many a middle-aged male at class reunion time.

With our own children in the highly impressionable stage, Karen has strongly hinted that I put the brakes on introducing some of my greatest childhood, teenaged and so-called grown-up male achievements to yet another generation.

I have politely been asked to refrain from turning our garage into a manufacturing depot for clothes pin match guns, tennis ball cannons, balsa wood bombers (with or without firecracker attached) or any of the other mishap-causing, dial 911 stuff that falls under the exasperated heading of boys will be boys.

It also was suggested that I probably should not inform youthful readers of the exact sciences involved in any of the above-listed mayhem makers. Better they should simply download hydrogen bomb instructions off the Internet.

He Learned It From His Father

I also was asked to not regale our children with Hardy Boy-like stories of the day I walked several miles of storm sewer under the city of Eau Claire, Wisconsin to find out for myself if it did, indeed, empty into algae-infested Half Moon Lake. It did and I would later lead entire expeditions of neighborhood kids along the same tennis shoe-soaking route, pointing out items of archeological interest such as the long-ago graffiti where Marsha apparently loved David.

Let's just say that sloshing along a stretch of salamander-infested storm sewer is not the career path usually mapped out by moms for their children. (See Above: really neat versus just plain stupid).

As for passing along the nuances of "mumbletypeg", Karen didn't even like the sound of it, much less the description.

In this day and age, when possession of a butter knife is enough to get a child suspended from elementary school until he or she is old enough to vote, the mere thought of a playground game involving hordes of jackknife-wielding school boys is enough to send most teachers' unions calling for the recess-time assistance of the National Guard.

According to at least one version of Webster's New World Dictionary, mumbletypeg is "a game in which a jackknife is tossed in various ways to make it land with the blade in the ground."

Although I am not 100 percent sure of the rules (nor was anyone else I asked in the interests of parenting-book accuracy), I do remember that mumbletypeg involved a degree of difficulty, with the jackknife being flipped from various fingers, forearms, elbows, knees and foreheads with the simple goal of sticking it in the dirt.

Many was the unfortunate Cub Scout who limped off the playground, his black Ked bearing the slash of a misplaced mumbletypeg flip.

Suffice to say, Tyler and Colin will not be participating in the national mumbletypeg championships, even if ESPN2 does run out of truck pulls. Between Karen and Hayley and their female sense of propriety, the boys will be lucky if they get away with one, "Pull my finger." But, even that would be really neat.

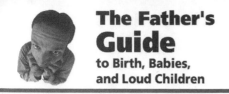

Chapter Seven

Keep Your Fingers To Yourself

According to many experts, or at least two of my friends who watch Oprah, most teachers strongly advocate parental involvement in the educational process.

Although this may be the politically correct public offering, savvy educators who speak with the weary voice of experience caution academic newcomers with one bit of sage advice.

"Be careful what you wish for. You may actually get it." This is said with the straight-faced sincerity that can only be mustered by someone joyfully skipping toward the door of early retirement.

With our children fully immersed in their pre-Ivy League curriculum of elementary school and pre-school, we are now among the army of the parentally involved, rallying behind the daily cry of, "Hurry up, you're going to be late for school."

In addition to time actually spent in the classroom, the commitment required by other school-related activities is staggering. In the first two months of the school year, extracurricular activities include such things as Girl Scouts, story night, potluck dinners, Parent Teacher Organization, wrapping paper sales, field trips, open house, snack day, parent-teacher conferences and Dad's Day.

There also were two things in which the students were expected to participate.

Like most parents new to the academic lifestyle, we were totally unprepared for the amount of nightly homework, none of which is actually done by the children.

Each night, the kitchen table is cluttered with reams of multi-colored forms and flyers requiring immediate attention as well as parental signatures. Somewhere in the stack is a signed permission slip giving ourselves permission to sign permission slips.

As with any endeavor, some of the bring-this-home-to-your-parents assignments are more enjoyable than others.

Such as the Mystery Box.

He Learned It From His Father

The Mystery Box was a staple of our children's preschool environment, brought home first by Hayley and then inherited by Tyler.

Each week, as the class works on learning a new letter, the Mystery Box is sent home with a student. The assignment, at least for most letters, is simple – put an object that starts with the weekly letter in the box and then write out a list of clues. The students, in a hand-waving frenzy, then try to guess what's inside the box.

For the letter "A," for example, an apple is put inside the Mystery Box, and the list of clues includes such stumpers as "It's red and grows on trees."

When Tyler brought home the Mystery Box for the letter "F," I immediately recalled one of my dad's all-time favorite tricks, which involved a hand-sized cardboard box with a hole cut in the bottom. The inside of the box was filled with gauze, colored red with iodine. My dad would then stick his finger through the hole in the bottom of the box. When he opened the lid, it looked exactly like a bloody chopped-off finger lying on the gauze. My sisters and I, of course, thought this was prop comedy at its finest. My mother thought otherwise.

As I laughingly tried to explain Grandpa's finger-in-the-box trick to Hayley, Tyler and Colin, I realized that a demonstration was in order. On short notice, I was forced to use ketchup instead of iodine, but the effect was the same.

The kids thought it was prop comedy at its finest. Karen, like most mothers and wives, thought otherwise.

She also did not think it overly wise to adapt the Mystery Box to accommodate the finger trick. She was probably right, but it was a shame to waste the well-thought out clues.

"When a driver cuts Mom off on a busy street, she gives him the (blank)."

"When you pull up at a stoplight, the man driving the other car usually has his (blank) in his nose."

"At a family reunion, your uncle says, 'Pull my (blank).'"

83

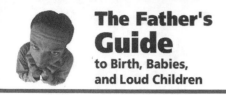
Chapter Seven

The whole thing turned out to be moot as Tyler actually had the letter "G."

When I picked up Tyler from preschool that day, I kiddingly told the teacher about the finger-in-the-box concept. I was surprised when her face brightened with recognition and she said, "My dad had one of those boxes." I took that as a sign of teacher-approved vindication.

I'm eagerly awaiting Colin's pre-school shot at the Mystery Box, hoping he is lucky enough to draw the letter "W." I know there's a whoopee cushion around our house somewhere. Hey, at least I'm involved.

The School of Hard Nyuks

When it comes to exposing children to fine art and culture, there are three things purposely ignored by females in general and mothers in particular.

Those three things are, of course, Larry, Moe and Curley.

For some strange eye-poking, hammer-bonking reason, *The Three Stooges* always have attracted a male-dominated audience. As with most lessons learned by males, this one was learned the hard way.

Before we were married, I invited my wife on a date that involved a *Three Stooges* film festival. A more perceptive person would have recognized the forced smile. Then again, a more perceptive person wouldn't have been dragging a member of the opposite sex whom he hoped to impress to an evening of Stooge mania.

Before Moe had whacked anyone with even one single, solitary board, I noticed a deep, rhythmic breathing from the next theater seat. While the Three Stooges beat, bounced and bashed each other across the silver screen, Karen blissfully settled into a sound, Stooge-free sleep.

Later, she simply said she didn't want to hurt my feelings. Besides, she needed the rest.

From that point on, my Stooge watching was limited to those early-morning or late-night occasions when their all-too-rare television appearances coincided with the few occasions where I was either home or in the office alone.

He Learned It From His Father

In one blast of black-and-white celluloid enlightenment, however, my favorite trio made a pre-breakfast reappearance into our lives to the delight of the kids.

For the most part, our children's exposure to TV is limited, restricted usually to classic Disney movies on video or some sort of child-friendly show on public television. Under the theory that nostalgic parents result in nerdy kids, they also think it's a great treat on Saturday nights to watch reruns of the old hokey-but-harmless *Lawrence Welk Show*.

In order to keep the house somewhat quiet on an early Saturday morning, I offered to let the two oldest, Hayley and Tyler, watch TV so mom and Colin could maybe get another hour of sleep.

With juice glasses in hand, they settled onto the living room pillows while I flipped through channel after channel of unsuitable programming.

Just as I was about to force them to watch the Weather Channel, one more click of the remote brought the pie-in-the-face slapstick comedy of *The Three Stooges* onto the screen.

Settling onto another pillow, I began to explain the premise of *Three Stooges'* humor to Hayley and Tyler, who stared at the TV in utter disbelief.

Talk about quality time. This was hands-on parenting at its finest. In between my own bursts of out-loud laughter, I was the wizened purveyor of a wealth of Stooges trivia. To my great delight, Hayley and Tyler were like sponges, soaking up the important basics like how the Curley episodes were vastly superior to those featuring Shemp and how a mixing bowl could be used for a Moe haircut.

For the future delight of teachers and classmates, they quickly had Curley's legendary phrases and antics down pat.

"Ah, wiseguy, eh? ... look at the grouse ... nyuk, nyuk, nyuk."

The patter was, of course, accompanied by bashing each other with pillows. Not Hayley and Tyler. Me and Hayley and then me and Tyler.

Unfortunately, the premise of quietly watching TV to allow Karen extra sleep evaporated when our gales of laughter awakened her and Colin.

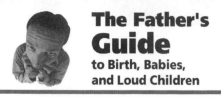
Chapter Seven

As she groggily, and somewhat angrily, asked from the bedroom what were we laughing about, Tyler raced in to the bedroom and proudly said, "Mom, dad let us watch the *Two Students*."

His shortcomings in math further added to the confusion. As he tried to explain what we had been watching, he finally blurted out, "You know, with Moe and Curley."

Hayley added to the review.

"Mom, it was so funny. They hit each other with pipes and sticks and they tried to pull the one with the funny hair cut through the wall."

The look on Karen's face let me know that this would probably be an item for future discussion.

Based on their initial reaction to *The Three Stooges*, or at least my perception of it, I have continually added to the curriculum of comedy education in our household.

One cross-county drive was accompanied by a five-video set of *The Little Rascals*. To battle Nebraska boredom, the kids loudly accompanied Alfalfa on "My Darling Clementine." In fact, they have picked things up so quickly, I think they may be ready for the Marx Brothers.

Putting The Chrome In Chromosome

I must have missed the automotive part of the maternity ward instructions.

"Congratulations! It's a boy. Gentlemen, start your engines."

From the first day of his first anything – first noise, first crawl, first fall down the stairs – Tyler has been turning our house into his version of a child-sized suburban truck stop.

Red trucks, blue trucks, black trucks, plastic trucks, wooden trucks, metal trucks, imaginary trucks, truck books, truck stickers, truck pajamas. The availability of truck underwear was the single motivating factor in leaving diapers in the dust. Yet, as near as we can determine, there is no rhyme or 18-wheel reason for this over-the-road mentality.

My own automotive aptitude is limited to the toll-free number on the back of my AAA card. My firsthand familiarity with truck stops is pretty much restricted to the occasional late-night bowl of roadside chili in GodKnowsWhere, USA and a long-standing, if somewhat less-than-public, fondness for songs such as "Six Days On The Road" and "Truck Drivin' Man."

From Tyler's standpoint, he has never participated in a father-and-son, don't-tell-your-mother-I-said-that, oil-changing session in our driveway. He has never been privy to repair work that required anything more than duct tape or a coat hanger. Karen's truck-driving resume consists primarily of thousands of child-hauling, stress-inducing minivan miles, which is not the stuff of jukebox favorites.

Hayley, like most little girls, has spent her time skipping down the traditional path of dress-up, Disney movies, Barbie dolls and big-sister bossiness.

As soon as Colin's truck-like noises started coming out of his mouth instead of the other end, he was on his hands and knees alongside Tyler pushing anything with wheels.

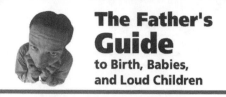

Chapter Seven

Despite this genealogical lack of diesel DNA, Tyler has been fascinated with trucks since Day One. He showed no interest in crawling until he discovered he could push a toy truck along in front of him, accompanied, of course, by the non-stop vroooom-vroooom-vroooom of an infant truck engine.

Accompanied, of course, by the non-stop vroooom-vroooom-vroooom of an infant truck engine and the non-stop vroooom-vroooom-vroooom of an infant truck engine and the non-stop vroooom-vroooom-vroooom of an infant truck engine.

As his actual vocabulary developed, the aforementioned vrooming noises were systematically replaced by carefully enunciated baby words such as da-da, ma-ma and Pe-ter-bilt.

Tyler also is quick to share his interest and knowledge of the diesel-truck industry. On any family outing, he is quick to loudly point out, "Look, there's a big truck," as we minivan our way across country.

On our last claustrophobic family trip to Florida, Tyler quickly and loudly pointed out, "Look, there's a big truck," some 47,374 times.

For his third birthday, we took him to the local Peterbilt dealer, where a very kind salesperson took the time to let Tyler and Hayley sit in the cab, raise the driver's seat up and down, blow the horn and turn on the windshield wipers. I'm afraid reading, 'riting and 'rithmetic may face some stiff competition in years to come.

In fact, Tyler already has narrowed his choices in higher education to either Harvard or the diesel truck driving school of his choice. Well, maybe an Ivy League school is the hoped-for destination of his overly optimistic parents, but mailing in the matchbook cover for truck-driving school is all Tyler's idea.

With our own background in diesel-engine maintenance sorely lacking, we have yet to figure out the source of the boys' fascination with trucks. Then again, we're not going to worry about it. We'll probably just keep on truckin'.

The Monsters Of Culture

In the snack-populated world of daily parenting, I must admit that the mention of "Newton" now triggers thoughts of cookies rather than classrooms. Fig has replaced Sir Isaac as the Newton of recognition.

As a refresher course, Isaac Newton was the cerebral half of the pre-vaudeville comedy duo, the Newton Brothers, and the inventor of gravity. The other, lesser-known brother, Groucho Newton, was, of course, the inventor of levity, which to this day forms the foundation of most father-child relationships.

One of our dad-and-kids Saturdays emphasized that most family outings are based on Sir Isaac's Law of Motion, "For every act of sophistication, there is an equal and opposite reaction of tackiness."

With all three of our kids home during a holiday break and insufficient snow to sentence them to 10-hour days of sledding, the pressure to maintain both childhood interest and parental sanity was intense.

As many moms are apt to do, Karen came up with an enlightened excursion, at least by our standards, of a trip to the museum.

It was great. The kids charged from exhibit to exhibit, soaking up information for use later in life as part of the play-along-at-home, TV game show audience. Throw in the museum-run old-fashioned candy shop and it was probably as much fun as learning allows.

Unfortunately, the cultural carry over of the museum trip lasted about as long as a commercial for sugar-coated cereal. By morning, the rallying cry was, "What are we going to do today?"

It was now my turn to plan and carry out the next minivan mission. Because we had been culturally elevated by our museum trip, I opted for the opposite end of the entertainment spectrum. The Thunder Nationals Monster Truck Show.

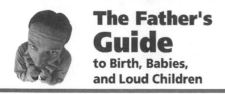

Chapter Seven

The kids greeted the choice with rampant enthusiasm and cheers of excitement. Karen greeted the choice by staying home alone with Home and Garden TV.

First, let me explain that I am not an avid motor sports fan. I shudder at radio commercials that scream, "SUNDAY!! SUNDAY!! SUNDAY!!" over the taped accompaniment of revving engines.

I always believed that if I went to a tractor pull or monster truck rally, and liked it, I would move all the kitchen and laundry appliances out to the front yard.

My own reservations were balanced by the desire to expose our children to as many things as possible under the theory that my gearhead prejudices should not automatically be theirs.

I am still not quite sure what it was we sat through, although Tyler and Colin cheered wildly as gigantic trucks named "Rambo" and "The Devastator" repeatedly drove over a row of already-flattened automobiles. At other times, a single monster truck would thunder down the hockey rink-sized concrete floor, stop and, with engines roaring and oversized tires smoking, spin wildly around in circles as Tyler and Colin encouraged them at the top of their lungs.

To her intellectual 7-year-old credit, Hayley mostly yawned and rolled her eyes through the whole deafening ordeal.

Intermission thrills were added when miniature cars and trucks zoomed in and raced around like demented parade Shriners. Our entertainment value was increased by the motorcyclist who roared in as if pursued by police and jumped over four, count 'em four, monster trucks and the woman who was shot out of a truck-mounted cannon.

Thanks to Isaac Newton and gravity, she landed safely in a drooping net at the far end of the arena. Thanks to Groucho Newton and levity, I can actually laugh about the fact that I paid money to see it.

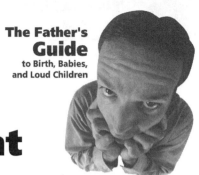

Chapter Eight

Home Sweet Home

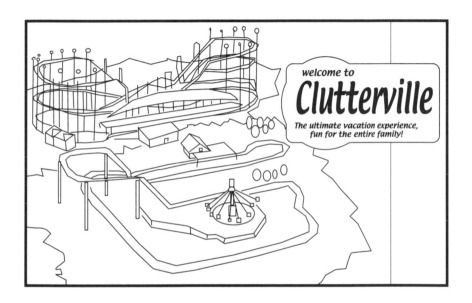

welcome to

Clutterville

The ultimate vacation experience,
fun for the entire family!

An Offer You Can't Refuse

Organized crime could learn a subtle thing or two from the purveyors of child safety products.

According to research, in this instance mostly late-night cable movies, the mob's protective services division generates suitcases full of unmarked revenue through its simple pay-or-else program, at least until the feds swoop in.

And, although everybody on 17 movie channels is threatened with bodily harm on a nightly basis, in reality I think their marketing strategy reaches a very small portion of the American public.

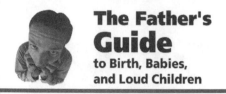
Chapter Eight

While Hollywood would have you believe people are literally dying to write M-A-F-I-A on the "pay-to-the-order-of" line of their next personal check, our household has never received a single catalog or direct-mail brochure (not counting political donations) suggesting we extortion-proof our home.

The child safety gang is another matter, however, relying on the time-tested selling points of guilt and fear. On a daily basis, stoop-shouldered postmen deliver the message, staggering under the collective four-color, high-gloss weight of dozens of mail-order catalogs, each hammering home the point that everything in your house is out to get your kids.

Of course, they're right. After docile decades of non-adult threatening existence, every nook, cranny, step, stair or pattern in the carpet suddenly is a potential hazard waiting and willing to grab the nearest unsuspecting child in mid-crawl.

Capitalizing on that parental paranoia, an entire industry has evolved around what magazine covers routinely, if somewhat incorrectly, refer to as, "child-proofing your home."

Actually, this is somewhat of a misnomer. The only true method of child-proofing a home is a massive titanium padlock on the front door that prohibits children from entering. Once a child is actually inside, however, the battle is on, every minute of every day, especially at our house, Casa de Kidtrap.

Our house, which makes Tom Hanks' purchase in *The Money Pit* look like a prudent investment, is somewhat strange (layout, not occupants, although that's a topic for discussion). The downstairs originally housed a window-making shop with the living quarters upstairs. Except for the clutter and no windows to sell, it's still the same. Everything is upstairs, including the kitchen and three kids who would prefer to be down stairs at all costs.

Pages 31, 32 and 33 of the catalog listed the child gates, which judging by the price were not only effective, but gold-plated. With safety a primary concern, however, the money was willingly paid without a threat from a single hoodlum.

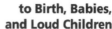

Home Sweet Home

The rest of the upstairs was a total disaster from the standpoint of child safety. Until she was 3 years old, Hayley thought her nickname was "Get Down," while Tyler, lovingly answered to "Don't Put That In Your Mouth." Nicknames aside, electrical outlets, cupboard doors, knife drawers, drapery cords, table corners and whatever else you could name had to be fixed.

Fortunately for us, the catalog person at the business end of the toll-free number was more than happy to accept our credit card number and, oh yes, two-day delivery was just an extra eight dollars.

One magazine article suggested that parents crawl around on their hands and knees to get a child's-eye view of potential hazards. The first time we did this, it immediately produced a big clump of dog hair near my right knee, which Tyler promptly picked up and, with the handspeed of David Copperfield, jammed into his mouth.

According to the catalogs, no room is more dangerous than the bathroom. Safety mats, faucet covers, water temperature indicators all are available for a pricey price. Another gadget called the "Lid Lock" was advertised under the headline, "Avoid the danger of an open toilet seat." Although most men eventually learn that the hard way, like say in the first week of marriage, installing the lock now might prevent spending the $80 the plumber charges after doll swimming lessons.

And that's the best thing about the whole child safety product industry – kids are willing conspirators. No matter how much child-proofing is done, it's never finished. When one thing is covered, another's discovered.

Fortunately, we just received our newest safety catalog. This one has a saggy-jowled Marlon Brando on the cover, making us a child-proof offer we can't refuse.

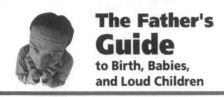
Chapter Eight

Earth To Martha Stewart

Just once I'd like to see Martha Stewart knee-deep in kid-based reality.

The entire premise of Martha's color-coordinated lifestyle of perfection is not based on money to spend or time to burn. Her ability to churn out an endless stream of gourmet meals with one hand while redecorating the kitchen with the other is based entirely on one fact and one fact alone.

There are no small children in the home-improvement world of Martha Stewart.

As the rest of us gamely battle the daily flood of toddler-inspired natural disasters, Martha nonchalantly goes about her televised business of brightening our lives, flitting from one pastel project to the next, unimpeded by the non-stop stampede of tiny feet.

While endlessly expounding on the virtues of pleated drapes, Martha strolls confidently through a spotless living room left over from the set of the *Donna Reed Show*, knowing full well she will never trip over a toy or have to embarrassingly explain a crayon-scribbled wall.

She never once has to rely on her version of the time-tested battle cry of the constantly interrupted, "STOP IT!!! CAN'T YOU SEE I'M TALKING TO MILLIONS OF PEOPLE!!!

In other words, she operates in that child-free universe known as La-La Land.

With three kids under the age of seven in our house, *Star Trek* is much closer to reality than is Martha Stewart.

Thanks to Hayley and her younger brothers, Tyler and Colin, our living room bears more of a resemblance to a war-torn global hot spot than it does to a showcase suitable for a national television audience.

If Martha had not gone to the bathroom by herself in seven years, she would not be so quick to use the phrase, "something to do when you have a little extra time on your hands."

Very rarely does Martha pick up an embroidered throw pillow, only to discover a long-forgotten bottle of now-curdled milk.

Home Sweet Home

When color-coordinating your outfit means hoping the prune stain on your shirt goes well with your sweet potato-spattered pants, you are not the audience targeted by Martha's sponsors.

And, I bet Martha never lost a load of laundry.

We did.

I'm not talking about the occasional sock that disappears from the dryer or a misplaced mitten. I'm talking about an entire load of laundry. That's right, an entire load, gone for three days.

As with the plot of any good whodunit mystery, the disappearance was not immediately noted. It was not until a desperate search failed to turn up a single piece of clean underwear for the kids that we realized something was amiss, even by our standards.

We searched every room in the house. Every bed was looked under, every closet emptied. Because a plastic trash bag occasionally was used to quickly and discretely transport laundry through the house when unexpected company arrives, we even checked the garbage cans in case a bulging black Hefty bag had been misdelivered.

Family meetings were held and individual members were asked to retrace their steps. Had somebody pilfered the pile piece-by-piece from the dryer as needed? Nope, not one single shred of clothing was in household circulation.

We were just about ready to put our laundry on the side of a milk carton when Karen noticed a familiar-looking sock partially peeking out from under a pile of something, which was mostly obscured by an unpacked suitcase, which was almost completely hidden from view by a push toy.

Not wanting to spook the long-sought underwear, we cautiously approached from the side, gingerly lifting the suitcase to reveal the freshly laundered Treasure of the Three-Cycle Kenmore.

As the family celebration commenced, I could not help but notice that the random colors of the hodgepodge pile of laundry went extremely well with the pattern in the rug and nicely brought out the beige in an almost-faded carpet stain. It was interior decorating at its finest.

Martha Stewart would have been proud of us.

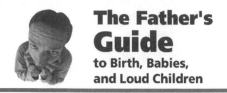
Chapter Eight

Bless This Mess

With one painfully honest childhood observation, we once elevated household clutter to the status of tourist attraction.

In the midst of a boisterous toddler-trashed morning, our daughter, Hayley, paused in mid-pileup long enough to answer the front door and greet our neighbor with a cheerful, "Hi. Do you want to come in and see our big mess?"

Although better judgment and an overall disdain for natural disasters normally would have driven our neighbor back down the driveway, the fact that she was there to pick up her own 3-year-old son forced her to accept the invitation to wade into the wreckage.

Even by our daily living room-in-shambles standards, this mess was huge, a CNN-type mother of all messes. And, one of which Hayley, her younger brother, Tyler, and their visiting co-conspirator, Carter, were immensely proud.

Under the guise of playing the official kid-version of "Big Wind Storm" (not to be confused with the Washington political version), the three of them had transformed our living room and all of its mismatched contents into the shattered aftermath of a post-tornado trailer park.

Every pillow in the house was piled high atop the coffee table, while a trail of couch cushions directed visitors to an overturned kiddie car. The couch itself was buried under a mountain of stuffed animals, topped by what appeared to be a heaping helping of every doll in the western hemisphere. A giant dustball of unknown origin was thrown in for good measure.

It was as if a Toys-R-Us store had exploded in our living room.

For good measure, the pint-sized pile makers added sound effects, standing in the middle of the devastation and rattling full-size sheets of newspaper to make as much noise as humanly possible.

The three of them were beaming with stereotypical pride as Hayley asked with all seriousness, "What do you think of the mess?"

Home Sweet Home

Unless you are well-schooled in urban renewal, few questions are tougher to answer off the top of your head.

As our neighbor politely oohed and aahed at the sheer magnitude of the stacked-up tonnage, it occurred to me that we may have inadvertently stumbled over a pile and onto a theme park idea of immense parental proportions.

Clutterville. The ultimate vacation experience, fun for the entire family.

Children under the age of five would be free to climb the fabric-softened mountains of Laundry Land, jumping from one unfolded pile to the next. Exciting prizes offered to the winner of the daily find-the-car-keys scavenger hunt.

Kids of all ages could tiptoe through the Scattered Toy Obstacle Course. Adults would receive 10 extra points for a stubbed toe, 20 points for an actual broken one. Two points would be deducted for each swear word.

Elementary school children could conduct an old-fashioned paper drive from the safety of the living room from season-long stacks of football-related sports pages. The annual Easter egg hunt would be conducted with the help of a dozen life-sized dust bunnies.

In the interest of fair play and sportsmanship, however, children of congresspersons would be prohibited from taking part in "Big Wind Storm."

Despite my visions of Disney-like riches, the look of shock on our neighbor's face forced me to reconsider.

Rather than rent a bulldozer, I opted for the book-on-tape version of "How to Organize Your Life & Get Rid of Clutter," which contained "scores of tips and techniques to bring order to your life."

Before I could give the cassette a quick listen and de-clutter our house, the tape disappeared beneath a pile of something or other. I'm sure it's around here somewhere. Until then, do you want to come in and see our mess?

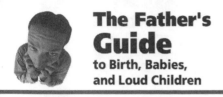
Chapter Eight

The Laundry Quandary

In the topsy-turvy, ever-changing wardrobe world of daily parenting, there is one reassuring constant that can be counted on without fail.

Laundry.

Clean or dirty, it is always present in some way, shape or form, hovering on the fringes of everyday life like an avalanche in waiting, ready to bury everything in its path under a blanket of whiter whites and brighter brights.

In a house with three children, ages 7, 6 and 3, the mathematical formulas for calculating daily laundry tonnage are simple, yet staggering.

The basic start-the-day attire of two socks, one underwear, one shirt, one pants is a straightforward five items per person.

With three children and two adults, that's 25 hamper-filling items per day. One basic washing machine load and one crock of mathematical hooey.

By the end of breakfast, spillage has claimed at least one of the children's outfits necessitating another trip to the closet, where, according to the laws of fashion, nothing matches.

The frenzied hunt for a coordinated outfit ultimately results not only in tears, but a bonus toss of at least one clean item of clothing directly into the basket of dirty clothes.

The laundry pile is bolstered by the half-dozen or so rags and towels used to clean up whatever part of the mess is not absorbed by a pair of khaki pants legs.

What breakfast and the ensuing argument failed to claim in terms of clean clothes is taken care of by a morning of nothing more than playing outside.

Although there hasn't been a cloud in the sky for the previous two weeks, our children manage to find a mud puddle on a daily basis.

The unwritten laws of kiddom require that anyone under the age of 10 has to wade into the middle of the puddle, regardless of footwear. Kids under the age of three are required to fall in it.

No tree is worth climbing unless its branches are covered with sticky sap and no bush is worth crawling under unless it is full of red, black or blue stain-producing berries

Home Sweet Home

By mid-morning, each of our three children is almost assuredly in outfit No. 2, pushing the daily clothing total to around 40 items, not counting rags and towels.

School-age children also are required at some point each day to change into and out of the proverbial school clothes.

Although I'm a bit fuzzy on the exact rules, little girls also are allowed at least one hysteria-induced, after-school changing session per week because Brittany or Heather or Jessica was wearing purple or pink or blue.

There also is some sort of "he, she or they are stupid" factor that enters into play, but is only understood by the first four rows of Bus 55.

Two more meals each day drastically increase the chance of another wardrobe accident, depending on the menu. Giving our children a plate of spaghetti has the same effect on their attire as telling them to lie down in a hog trough.

Weather also has a significant impact on laundry baskets. In many areas, the only thing that changes more often than the weather is the wardrobe needed to keep up with it. Northern winter weather requires two complete additional layers of clothing – one under and one over – with the end result being three soaking wet layers of clothes that require changing into a dry fourth set and another round of towels.

Any recreational activity or sport of any kind is carte blanche to bring home as many dirty, sweaty, damp clothes as you can fit into one sports bag.

The day usually is capped off by another towel-required bath or shower, followed by a pair of pajamas, possibly with an undershirt.

The next day and the next day and the next day after that, the process is repeated. We have been told by veteran parents (who have gone through three or four washing machines) that the laundry cycle usually lasts about 18 years, except for kids coming home from college.

Once the day's accumulation of laundry is finally put to rest, mathematics once again conspires to make one thing perfectly clear.

There is no truth to the phrase, "I'm done with the laundry."

According to laundry room guidelines, a dryer of any kind must take exactly twice as long per load as the washing machine. Even when you get ahead, you're behind. And, our kids are outside in a puddle.

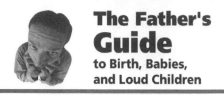
Chapter Eight

Mr. Fixit Wrecks His Dream House

Despite a half-century head start, Slippery Eddie, the Prince of Plywood, has proven to be no match for our kids.

According to local legend, Slippery Eddie was the nickname given to the contractor who built our house some 50 years ago. This was, of course, laughingly explained to us by elderly neighbors just after the ink had dried on the closing papers.

When first built, the ground level of what is now our house was used as a window-making shop, while the upstairs contained the living quarters. At the time, Slippery Eddie and his crew apparently hammered away under one consistent philosophy: "You can never use too many nails."

Slippery Eddie's love for anything "built in" has revealed itself over the years as a 10-penny roadblock firmly standing in the face of any attempted remodeling. Cabinets were securely nailed to wooden backs, which in turn were securely nailed to another layer of wood, which was nailed through to more wood and the whole thing then re-nailed into a wooden wall.

The house, as they say, was solid. Until our children were born. Since then our entire house and all of its contents have been dismantled, dented, dinged, bent, broken, spilled, split, pulled open, pried apart, torn, trashed and, for good measure, thrown up on. We are probably one correctly filled out government form away from federal aid.

Under the energized rules of "we're just playing," Hayley and Tyler roar through the house like a pair of jump-suited hurricanes, leaving an accidental wake of disaster and destruction. Advertising terms such as unbreakable, shatter-proof and stain resistant are little more than marketing myths. The Gray-Hoehn law of childhood physics is simply, "Anything that can be broken, will be broken."

Home Sweet Home

Drawer knobs that have withstood five decades of adult tugging, thanks to 12 layers of phlegm-colored enamel, magically pop off with the gentle pull of a 2-year-old hand. Toys carefully chosen to avoid choking are perfect for stopping up a 50-year-old drain, then slowly working their way through 50-year-old plumbing before firmly lodging themselves behind a 50-year-old cabinet, which is securely nailed to wooden backs, which are securely nailed to...

Requests for replacement parts are referred to an 87-year-old, suspender-wearing hardware store veteran who invariably responds, "I haven't seen one of these in years." The life expectancy of tabletop furnishings is precisely predicted by the height of the soon-to-occur fall.

And, even though in our house we're not exactly talking about Ming vases, a shattered anything results in a torrent of 2-year-old tears, which can only be stopped by Dad's optimistic phrase, "We can fix that."

Which is nice except for the fact that despite my claim, intentions and best efforts, I can't fix anything.

But that doesn't stop me from trying.

Armed with a tube of glue, a roll of tape and a gun full of staples, the great repair project gets underway. Piece A is connected to Piece B, this goes here, this gets stuck on this, that goes over there, and, Voila! Good as new.

Two hours later when the kids are, in theory, fast asleep and the recently fixed whatever falls apart again, it is quietly swept into the trash according to the out-of-sight, out-of-mind school of unsuccessful home repair.

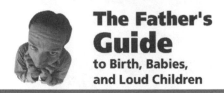
Chapter Eight

Not counting the overflowing water heater at midnight on a Saturday with a washer full of clothes and Tyler no longer full of diarrhea (which was almost *Three Stooges*-like in its comic unbelievability), the second most critical semi-attemptable home disaster was the sudden stoppage of Hayley's loud, obnoxious, beeping, buzzing, talking toy cellular phone.

After several thread-stripping attempts, the phone and its 43 pieces finally fell apart on my desk to reveal three small leaking batteries, which were simply replaced on a three-hour shopping trip to 14 stores.

With great perseverance, and an incredible amount of luck, the phone not only went back together, IT WORKED!!! For just nine dollars, two tanks of gas and one full day of labor, I had fixed a $2.99 toy telephone.

But, Hayley was ecstatic. Take that Slippery Eddie.

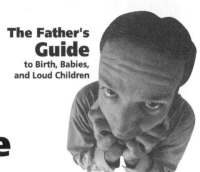

Chapter Nine

Mr. Mom

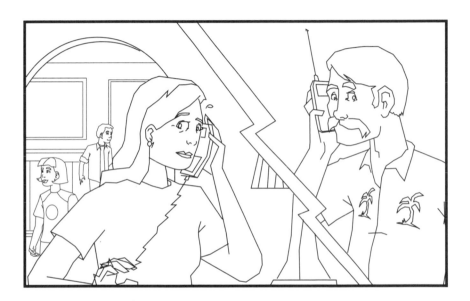

Mission Control,
We Have A Problem

The recipe for disaster in most homes is simple and consistent.
One parent leaves.

The who, what, when, where and why surrounding the departure is irrelevant. Whether it's a 10-minute trip to the grocery store or an overnight jaunt to anywhere blissfully quiet, the stay-behind parent is, as they say, in for it.

It is almost as if the ignition key in the obligatory minivan is linked directly to the family doom machine. One parent hops in the van, waves goodbye, cranks the stereo and backs down the driveway before the stranded parent has a change of heart.

Chapter Nine

A glance in the rearview mirror shows a forlorn wave accompanied by the facial expression of a *Titanic* passenger watching the last half-full lifeboat row off into the night.

Despite the tugging of heartstrings, common sense tells the parent on the verge of automotive freedom to put the pedal to the metal and deal with it later.

I know first-hand the trials and tribulations of a solo weekend with the kids.

My own first attempt at a stay-behind gig disintegrated in the face of an all-out assault by the flu and a puff of smoke from a burned-out furnace. The rebuilding of shattered confidence has been a slow and painful process. The mere sound of an opening garage door triggers a family-sized anxiety attack.

Since then, whenever I am on the road, I have a newfound appreciation for the telephone voice of exasperation.

Technology also has done wonders for the delivery of bad news.

There no longer is a five- or six-day delay while a heck-bent-for-leather pony express rider tracks down a traveling parent with news from home that one of the kids had toilet-papered another settler's mud hut, triggering a four-state range war.

Car phones, cell phones, pagers and e-mail now enable tales of family woe to be distributed immediately. By the same token, it makes it all but impossible to find peaceful sanctuary, far removed from the world of lost car keys, lost tempers and lost minds.

The days of leaving the phone off the hook or having the bartender relay the message, "He ain't here," have gone the way of quality TV programming.

Although many households simply are the site of occasional disaster, we actually have an entire period of catastrophe that coincides with the end of the high school basketball season.

As a sportswriter, the annual state basketball tournaments were my equivalent of what many males refer to as a "business trip." The very nature of the tournament required a three-day stay on successive weekends in our illustrious state capital, surrounded by dozens of other minivans, each of whose windows proclaimed in white shoe polish, "On To State."

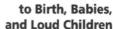

Mr. Mom

While I was knee-deep in stat sheets, scorebooks, empty coffee cups and Mighty Malt containers, Karen, was home knee-deep in... well, I don't want to actually know, but I'm sure she was knee-deep in something.

Each phone call home, even without the benefit of a comedian-inspired dial 10-10-hidden charges, hinted at an ever-increasing level of insanity.

Even by our level of disorganization, however, one state tournament weekend may finally have set a standard for Gray-Hoehn disaster that, like many great sports records, will never be broken.

As I was winding up my 27th adjective-free wire service basketball story, I made one last call to mission control to check in on how things went at home.

I should have known better.

As near as I could gather from Karen's stranger-than-true description, her home alone Saturday with Hayley, Tyler and Colin unfolded like this:

Couldn't find a babysitter. Office worker hadn't eaten. Put a pizza in the oven. Start macaroni and cheese for kids. Doorbell rings. Left kids alone at table. Ran to door. Neighborhood kids having a scavenger hunt. Found sought-after item. Ran upstairs. Start bathwater. Doorbell rang. Dog ran for door, got tangled up and pulled phone cord out of the jack. Phone bounced on floor, split into several pieces. Ran for the door. More neighborhood kids. More scavenger hunt. Put sign outside, "Please Do Not Ring Doorbell." Ran upstairs. Knocking at door. More knocking at door. Incessant knocking at door. Run downstairs. More kids. Shout upstairs, "Are you kids all right?" Worker calls. Newspaper missing basketball scores. Stop bathwater. Run downstairs. Smoke alarms go off. Run upstairs. Pizza cheese dripped, oven on fire. Put out fire. Macaroni boils over. Baby crawls for full-to-top bathtub. Rescue him. Deliver burned pizza to worker. Other than that things are OK.

It was as if I had left and the Marx Brothers moved in.

The good news is, when I got home, everything was, indeed, OK. The better news is that there are more tournaments ahead. I can hardly wait for the phone call.

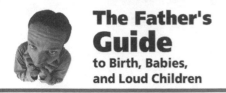

Chapter Nine

The Dangers Of Flying Solo

My deep appreciation for those in the stay-at-home trenches was both earned and learned the hard way.

Among all household disasters, nothing is as loud as the sound of shattered confidence. As most women will attest, there is a reason why many men take being called a "know it all" as the ultimate compliment. That is especially true when it comes to actually running the household. As every guy knows and is quick to point out, there is no way that staying home with one, two or three or more kids is nearly as difficult and demanding as sitting behind a desk for eight hours.

In terms of that attitude, I was guilty as charged until Karen went over the wall for the first time on a solo vacation sans children, spouse, dog and daily grind.

Her pre-trip excitement, which was quietly and calmly punctuated by the phrase, "I'M OUTTA HERE!!!" was somewhat offset by her concerns about leaving our kids home alone with yours truly.

From my perspective, how hard could it have been to handle two children, who at that time, were under the age of four for a mere five days?

Out of bed, breakfast, dressed, playtime, lunch, oldest to pre-school, youngest to nap, pick-up pre-schooler, dinner, baby sitter arrives, kids to bed.

I mean, come on, this was simple I'm-in-charge-parenting, not a shuttle launch. In other words, "Have a nice trip, we'll be fine."

I had even taken steps to overcome my own acknowledged shortcomings.

Based on my own complete indifference to daily attire (it's hard to mismatch jeans and a T-shirt), I was honest enough to request pre-trip assistance from the wardrobe department. As such, five sets of daily outfits were hung together and plainly labeled Saturday through Tuesday. I was guessing Hayley got the dresses.

All other contingencies were covered. Medicinal dosages for each and every sniffle, sneeze and tropical fever were spelled out to the nearest quarter teaspoon. Emergency telephone numbers, including the National Hurricane Center in Miami and the Butterball Turkey Hotline, were tacked inside the cupboard door.

Mr. Mom

The next morning, the stay-at-home delegation saw mom off at the airport with a deeply touching, heartfelt "Don't forget to bring us presents." I have a feeling any twinge of guilt Karen was feeling was absorbed as advertised by the two-across leather seating of Midwest Express airlines.

The difference between mom's approach and dad's way of doing things was quickly apparent. On the way home from the airport, four years of nutritional breakfasts were undone in one fast-food stop. (Hey, 20 years from now, doctors will still need patients.)

With the first grease-laden culinary battle behind us, we quickly settled in to our lack of routine.

Frozen pizzas literally became the order of the day. Pre-bedtime baths were replaced by early morning showers, complete with the cheerful, barracks-like admonishment of, "MOVE, MOVE, MOVE!!!! Dad has work to do." (As if mom never does.)

Actually, dad did have work to do, but based on my well-thought-out, mom's-gone planning, Hayley and Tyler would join me in the office and things would hum along as usual.

Two days later, I was two days behind in my work.

Other than that, we were, as confidently predicted, fine. A point that was emphasized and re-emphasized to mom on every one of her phone calls home. As we breezed through day four of our survival training, I realized I was within one day of being able to smugly say, "I told you so."

Less than 24 disaster-filled hours later, however, the white flag of surrender was flying above the compound. When Karen made her next phone call home, there was no hiding the panic in my voice.

"What's wrong?"

"Well, what do you want first, the good news or the bad news?"

She said it didn't matter and she was right. We had already hit the iceberg.

In brief it was . . .

BAD NEWS: The furnace went on the fritz, the repairman looked at it and laughed because that model had been recalled seven years ago. It has to be replaced immediately.

GOOD NEWS: The replacement furnace is free. All we have to pay for is installation.

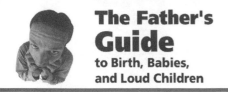
Chapter Nine

BAD NEWS: It will be a couple of days before we have heat.

To offset the lack of heat, I brought Hayley and Tyler into our bed. Tyler brought his flu germs. Two hours later, I remembered diarrhea as more than a trick word on spelling tests. I remembered spelling tests every 45 minutes or so for the rest of the night.

Tyler celebrated his crib-free sleep with a resounding THUMP! as he rolled off the side of the bed onto the hardwood floor. Hayley's screaming nightmare quickly diverted my attention away from Tyler. The trash man came at dawn and the dog promptly went berserk.

When Karen finally came through the front door, it was apparent the cavalry had arrived in the nick of time. We were out of ammunition, supplies and patience.

There are still times when I hear the door open and panic. As is often the case, she is the voice of reassurance. "It's OK, I'm just taking out the garbage."

It's a 17-second round trip. Don't worry. I've got everything under control.

Survivor: Our House

When it comes to acknowledging sheer marketing audacity, you have to tip your hat to the creative minds at CBS.

Armed with nothing more than a gazillion-dollar budget and an unshakable belief in the gullibility of a country that bought 30 million Chia Pets, the geniuses behind network TV convinced a prime time audience that 16 adults spending several child-free weeks in the Australian outback with a chance to win a million dollars somehow qualifies as risk-taking.

Like most parents whose only goal is to make it through the day, I was somewhat skeptical of how risky things actually were for the photogenic participants of the heavily hyped, "Survivor 2: The Australian Outback."

So, in the interest of editorial accuracy, I convinced Karen that I needed 60 uninterrupted minutes for television research. With the kids safely in the bath tub under her supervision, I escaped with the remote in an hour-long pursuit of serious journalism.

The premise of "Survivor" was simple. Sixteen of what the network cleverly referred to as, "average Americans, chosen from all walks of life" were dumped in the middle of the Australian Outback. Participants, dressed in resort casual, were split into two competing tribes that took part in a variety of games and contests that resembled spring break on "Gilligan's Island."

Every three days, the Survivors gathered to vote someone out of their respective tribe. In a solemn ceremony patterned after the "Thank you sir, may I have another," paddling in the movie *Animal House*, the back-stabbing Survivors banished their most obnoxious member with the haunting admonishment, "the tribe has spoken."

The dejected non-Survivor then trudged off to a never-ending stream of lucrative guest appearances on the TV talk-show circuit.

At the end, the lone survivor won one million dollars without having to face Regis Philbin.

The biggest problem faced by participants, other than their personalities, was the daily hunt for food. Under the watchful eye of an official Crocodile Dundee-type Australian, tribal members consumed a variety of bugs, worms and other disgusting stuff, thereby proving something or other.

The rest of the on-air time was spent whining and complaining about other tribe members.

The quest for the million dollars was not without risk, however. One member's riveting account of another death-defying day on the outback was listed on the official Survivor 2 website.

"With less shade than at Kucha's beach and under a blazing sun for most of the day, Ogakor tended to be more lethargic than their opponents. 'We are more of a recreational tribe, we lie around a lot,' said Tina, the personal nurse from Tennessee. The tribe also liked to play at their 'whirlpool,' a shallow section of the river with light rapids that served as massage jets. Maralyn couldn't have put it any better: 'There is a time to be energized and a time to chill out, so we are going to the whirlpool.'"

In other words, these so-called Survivors wouldn't have lasted one afternoon in our house or any other house with children.

So in the interest of equal time and unlimited endorsement opportunities, we are proposing "Survivor: Our House" on behalf of beleaguered parents everywhere.

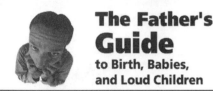
Chapter Nine

Participants, who assumed they would be spending a month or so in paradise, would instead be surprisingly dropped into a typical American home, complete with at least three children under the age of 7. As in real life, babysitters would not be available or would cancel at the last minute.

Food foraging would include the baby food challenge, where tribal members sample jar after jar of combined delicacies such as chicken-apple and liver-asparagus. Adult meals would consist of unmarked Tupperware leftovers.

The dual diaper change would provide a grueling test of breath-holding ability as one member simultaneously tackles the overflowing diapers of two infants while the third child attacks the dog food bin. As soon as the adult has one diaper in each hand, the phone rings with an all-important call from a not-to-be-denied telemarketer.

Ripping the phone from the wall is a two-hours-of-sleep penalty

The final round would simply be *The Great Escape*. On a given signal, remaining tribe members would bolt for the door. The lone survivor would be left behind to answer to the children.

"WE'RE HUNGRY. I HAVE TO GO TO THE BATHROOM. HE HIT ME FIRST. SHE STARTED IT. THE DOG THREW UP. I'M TELLING ON YOU. YOU STINK."

The tribe has spoken.

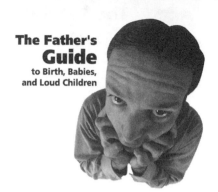

Chapter Ten

An Exercise
In Futility

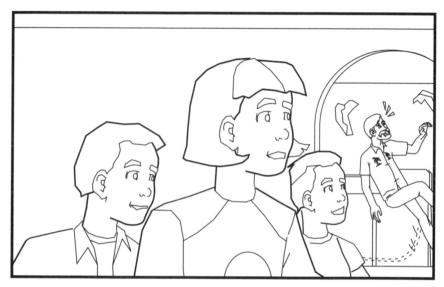

Workout With The KidMaster

With little fanfare and no color-coordinated Spandex, I have discovered the ultimate exercise program. Daily parenting.

Thanks to our children, I have three pint-sized personal trainers, fulfilling their demanding duty 24 hours a day, seven days a week, 365 days a year. From sunup to sundown, Karen and I are put through our paces, lifting, chasing and carrying.

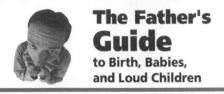
Chapter Ten

Loads of groceries, which probably should be delivered by rail car, are instead loaded bag by muscle-fatiguing bag into the minivan. Upon the return home, the entire back-breaking process is repeated in reverse, compounded by the fact that our kitchen at Rancho Poorly Designed is on the second floor. Our house is one gigantic sweat-producing StairMaster. Up, down, up, down, that's it, deep breaths, up, down, up, down.

Based on grocery industry standards, which require that one bag in three rip at the seams when packed with anything heavier than cotton balls, an entire sackful of something invariably ends up on the driveway. OK class, let's work on those deep-knee bends.

In a house with small children, there is no such thing as laundry day. They are all laundry days. Kids clothes are the sponges of the fashion industry.

If the kids walk within 50 feet of a puddle, their pants immediately soak up every drop of brown muddy water. Meal times are a sit-down, family style game of who can spill what. Every crayon, marker and colored pencil conspires to run or bleed into whatever clothing it can stain. The entire multi-colored collection is then heaped into laundry baskets that weigh as much as the governor of Minnesota and, of course, go back downstairs. Then upstairs. Then downstairs.

And this is just daily existence. This has nothing to do with the playtime demands of three energetic children whose primary idea of fun is to run. No destination, no direction, no specific anything. Just run. In fact, it's the kids equivalent of "Gentlemen start your engines."

At any given moment, in the middle of whatever, Hayley, Tyler and Colin look at one another and simply say, "Let's run." And they do. As with any in-tune family unit, Karen and I also look at each other and simply say, "You chase them." In spousal discussion, if you are slow to respond, you'd better be fast with your feet. To discourage some of the track meets, we have raised several doorknobs, latches and levers above their reach. As Dr. Benjamin Spock, the '60s baby guru, said, "Offense wins games, defense wins championships." When the kids were much smaller and more liftable, I mistakenly instituted

An Exercise In Futility

the game of double-carry, where I would grab them both in my arms like two more bags of groceries and carry them up the stairs, complete with fake huffing, puffing and the obligatory-but-untrue, "You're too heavy, I'm going to drop you." They thought this was great sport and would laugh hysterically all the way to the top.

Unfortunately, they now weigh a combined 90 pounds or so and still think the double-carry is the funnest of fun family traditions. Of course they also still believe the huffing, puffing and threats of being dropped are parental acting at its finest, although far from the out-of-shape truth.

A horizontal variation of the double-carry was a mid-winter sledding excursion where I laid down on a hard piece of purple plastic. Two of the kids piled on top of me and off we went. With each successive bump, my snowsuit-wrapped passengers bounced another breath of air out my flattened-out chest. Some 37 bounces later when we reached the bottom, I resembled a played-out accordion. The kids, of course, thought we should do it again immediately, but only if I would pull them both back up the hill.

Parental exercise is not, however, limited to lifting heavy objects. Sometimes grace and agility are required, although both are extremely rare among rugby players turned fathers.

On one occasion, while searching for one of my usual tacky T-shirts, I spotted one in a neatly folded laundry pile (someone must have broken into our house and done the laundry). I nonchalantly reached for the pile and the next thing I know I was whizzing across the hardwood floor, completely out of control, arms windmilling wildly as I tried to regain my balance before finally smashing into the edge of dresser. It was slapstick at its finest. As I limped to the kitchen and asked if, by chance, someone, anyone knew anything about something spilled on the floor, Hayley and Tyler proudly informed that it was a slippery lotion trap like they had seen in the remake of the *Parent Trap* movie.

They seemed genuinely concerned when I warned them of the dangers of such a stunt, although in reality I admired their ingenuity. When I said I was a little sore from the fall, they were extremely helpful. They told me I should get more exercise.

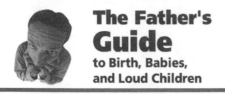
Chapter Ten

My Knees Need Kneading

If you divide 80 or 90 by two, then I guess I am what is known as a middle-aged father. Our three kids were born when I was between the ages of 40 and 45. The tradeoff is, in theory, you make up for lack of stamina with intelligence and experience. While the jury is still out on that one, certain activities point out the reality of the statement.

When Colin, our youngest, was in the learning to crawl stage, two ground-level laps around the recliner, made it painfully evident that I was four decades beyond the medal round of the toddler Olympics.

As with most kids whose actual first step is one step beyond their capability, Colin, settled into a daily exercise routine that consisted mostly of crawling through the entire house with surprising speed and an unsurprising lack of caution; a 30-pound wind-up toy with little sense of direction. Whether it was an outside surface of grass or dirt or any type of indoor flooring, the moment his bottom touched terra firma, he was off as if blasted out of an air cannon.

Unable to step over anything higher than a carpet pattern, his approach was much more ground-oriented, hugging the terrain like a sleeper-clad army tank as he rolled up and over pillows, toys and the family dog.

He rarely detoured, stopping only when he finally slammed head first into a wall, piece of furniture or the shin of an unsuspecting adult. On those occasions, he simply backed up, cleared his head and took off in the direction of another crawl-stopping obstacle.

Like many recreational enthusiasts, however, he quickly discovered that his passion was much more enjoyable when shared with others.

Although his older brother and sister occasionally would drop down to his level, it was evident that they could not usually be bothered with such childish antics. That is, unfortunately, where I crawled into the picture.

Colin was sitting by himself, surprisingly stationary and perfectly content while dismantling someone else's Lego project, when I made the mistake of dropping down to the floor, grabbing at him with both hands and giving him a the time-tested fatherly growl of the I'm-gonna-get-you monster.

An Exercise In Futility

Zoom, he was gone. Under the coffee table, over the dog, past the potted plant and behind the recliner, stopping only to peak back and see if he was being pursued. And, if not, why not. The chase, as they say, was on.

As I started crawling after him, he immediately shifted into high gear, shooting around the corner of the chair, squealing wildly with delight as I was left not only in the dust, but also the dog hair and Lego wreckage.

In the first foot and a half, the carpet had stripped away two layers of skin off each of my knees. Two crawls later, my right knee dropped painfully onto the blue-plastic booby trap of an upturned double Lego. As I sat up to pry the business end of the Lego out of my leg, I managed to attack the unarmed corner of the coffee table with my lower back.

As the game ground to a halt, Colin sat up and maniacally clapped his hands. It was painfully obvious that he was ready to go again, but more painfully obvious that I was not.

In talking with other battered and bruised parents, it was evident that Colin was not the only toddler to invent athletic events whose skill requirements precluded adult participation.

One of his favorite games was the handless, 360-degree spin. Taking advantage of the fact that 75 percent of his body weight was in his cheeks, facial and gluteal, he simply plopped onto his bottom and kicked his heels. With no other outward effort, he magically spun completely around as if his diaper contained its own Lazy Susan. Any parent who can do this is guaranteed a spot on David Lettermen.

Hayley and Tyler are not without their own athletic endeavors, each of which is guaranteed to pull at least one adult muscle.

Hayley is continually inviting me to swing upside down on the monkey bars or participate in the dips and dives, twists and turns of her self-choreographed dance program.

Tyler has encouraged me to follow him through kids-only bushes and shrubs where he duck walks under the overhanging branches of a 19-inch high evergreen. Visions of a fire department rescue and its accompanying newspaper account have kept me out of the arborvitae.

The return to childhood games has not been without its educational benefits. The jump from zero children to three has left us in dire need of a larger arena in the form of remodeling.

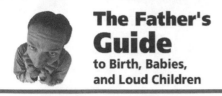

Chapter Ten

As an architect sat down to go over some preliminary plans for possible remodeling and expansion, he asked if we wanted a crawl space. No thank you. My knees already have all they can handle.

Ambush At Shallow End

Somewhere in the western wilds of suburbia, a parenting peer is gunning for the Lone Ranger of the West End YMCA.

More than three decades after my own towel-snapping days as a member of the Flying Fish class, I have found myself saddling up the trusty minivan for twice-weekly trips to the obviously misnamed "Y" for infant, toddler and children's swimming classes.

Although the first two letters of YMCA allegedly stand for "Young Men's," there are few other fathers, young or otherwise, holding in their stomachs in either swimming class. Despite the absence of a black swim mask, In most instances, I was the Lone Ranger – the only male over the age of three in the shallow end.

Which, of course, means I also am the only participating parent that emerges child-in-tow from the men's locker room.

When Tyler or Colin have swimming lessons, this is no big deal – a leisurely put your suit on, burp and occasional scratch, we belong here, father and son stroll through the chromosome comforts of jock-strap land.

Hayley, on the other hand, presented a slightly different problem, not just because of gender, but also because of her penchant for conversation. From the minute she could talk, Hayley was a chatterbox with no volume control and the observatory powers of a NASA satellite. As such, we jointly hustled through the men's locker room with one of us hoping and praying to avoid any and all anatomical question-and-answer sessions. The "No Running" rule did not apply until we hit poolside.

Despite being the only father in class, I was on almost equal footing once we were actually in the water. Just another harried and harassed, "What did I forget?" parent fervently hoping that it turns out to be someone else's child who goes to the bathroom in the pool.

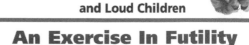
An Exercise In Futility

At times, however, I am still the unavoidable aquatic answer to the question, "What does not fit in this picture?" And, this is not in reference to the occasional cannonball. In this instance, I am referring to singalong time

With the fervor of a splash-happy tabernacle choir, parents and kids alike readily run through the entire repertoire of swim class favorites such as "The Hokey Pokey," "The More We Get Together," "Twinkle, Twinkle Little Star," and the ever-popular "Humpty Dumpty Sat On The Wall."

Possessing the only barroom baritone is a hard-to-hide distinction, especially among an entire pool full of lilting and cheery swim mother falsettos. At times it sounds as if the Von Trapp family suddenly had been joined by Johnny Cash, an off-key musical mismatch that echoes for hours off the tile-covered walls.

Not having an above-the-waist half of a swimming suit also can be a disadvantage, especially when the lifejacket, kickboard or foam noodle suddenly has shot from reach. In that instance, there is nothing like a huge handful of chest hair to grab, pull, and pull some more until panic subsides.

At times, I guess, I can actually hit those high notes.

Judging by one mid-class conversation, however, it appears as if I was no longer destined to be the only father in class.

As one little girl gamely tried to muster the courage to leap from the side of the pool, her mother nonchalantly pointed in my direction and said in her best co-conspirator voice, "See, your dad could bring you to swim class. There's another dad here. You'll have to tell him he wouldn't be the only one."

Right now, somewhere on a comfortable couch, some unsuspecting father is getting the business from an eager 2-year-old, his last feeble male excuse at avoiding swim class shot to pieces by the Lone Ranger.

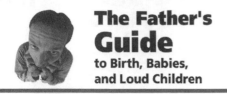
Chapter Ten

Babysitters, An Endangered Species

At the risk of stuck-at-home oversimplification, the blame for our lack of social life can be laid squarely at the sneaker-encased feet of women's sports.

The problem of parental house arrest is best summed up by what acronym-loving marketing types call the WNBA, or the Women's National Basketball Association.

For those of us whose last movie ticket cost $1.50, what the WNBA really stands for is, We're Not Babysitters, Anymore.

In other words, any female with enough athletic ability to keep up with three active children now is on a full-ride scholarship to someplace like Duke or Stanford or toting a gym bag full of sponsorships through an Olympic training camp.

For previous generations of let's-go-out-tonight parents, this type of award-winning athletic ability simply qualified high school- and college-age girls as in-demand babysitters.

Now, anyone whose Nike-swooshed athletic uniform conceals a sports bra is off running, jumping, swimming or skating from one event to another.

Any athletic attribute is a babysitting asset. Sprinter speed provides hope of corralling three bedtime-avoiding kids. Gymnastic flexibility reaches under the couch where no hand has gone before, into the universe of lost balls, wadded-up socks and the occasional forgotten sippy cup of old milk. Martial arts medalists simply stand a fighting chance of survival.

The 30-year exodus of every athletic Thomasina, Dixie and Harriet from home economics to the home team has made babysitters rarer than understandable song lyrics.

In some instances, babysitting also is apparently against the law.

As if messing up an entire country was not enough, Congress entered the fray on the side of athletic women and drained the entire babysitting pool thanks to something called Title IX of the Education Amendments.

An Exercise In Futility

Basically, Title IX mandates equal opportunity for men and women athletes at any school receiving federal funding. Although the Congressional legalese is a bit hard to decipher, I think it basically means that if you use the point guard on the women's basketball team as a babysitter, you can somehow get sued.

The on-court competition pales in comparison, however, to the battle for qualified babysitters.

With the odds of finding a sitter similar to those of being hit by lightning, claustrophobia and parental sanity demand that the search continue for that one smart, dependable person who not only can handle three children under the age of 7, but is willing to do so for less than $300 an hour.

No stone is left unturned. Relatives, friends, friends of friends, friends of relatives and seemingly trustworthy strangers are continuously pumped for babysitter leads.

In a creative moment of desperation, I once struck babysitter gold on the supermarket message board. Or so I thought.

When Karen was about eight months pregnant with our second child, I was making the daily grocery run for the hormone-induced craving of the moment when I happened to glance at the postcard-filled message board.

The bold, black letters of a fine point Sharpie were the parental equivalent of winning lotto numbers. "Bright, energetic 18-year-old looking to babysit."

This was obviously too good to be true. Based on the generation gap of TV viewing, my first instinct was to whirl around and look for Alan Funt and his Candid Camera, enjoying a nationwide joke on the gullible parent who, in a moment of desperation, actually fell for the unemployed babysitter stunt.

When no TV funnyman appeared, I discretely pocketed not only the phone number, but the entire postcard, rather than risk losing the prize to another stressed-out parent.

Chapter Ten

At the time, Karen was somewhat less than enamored with her appearance, using descriptive words like "schmarvy" and "schlumpfing." She was much less self-enamored when the 18-year-old, 6-foot-tall, blonde-haired, model-thin babysitter off the supermarket card showed up at our door. She did a wonderful job with the kids, but next time I will make sure the supermarket card contains key words such as frumpy, middle-aged and unattractive.

Thanks to an athletic group of neighborhood girls, we once again find ourselves in familiar territory. Sitter-less.

Sports and high school graduation have depleted our well-protected "A" list and the supermarket message well has run dry. So, we'll probably just stay home tonight and watch TV. I'm sure there's a women's basketball game on somewhere.

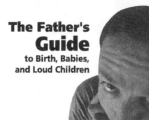

Chapter Eleven

Cool Cars:
A Thing Of The Past

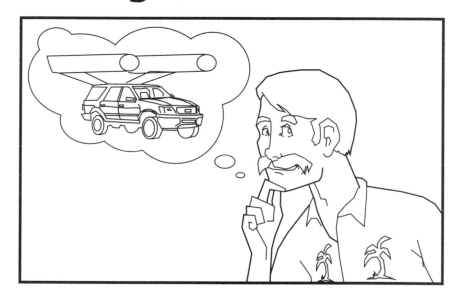

The Minivan Lifestyle

In the uncompromising, engine-revving world of automotive hipness, few things radiate total uncoolness like the stereotypical suburban minivan. Since the first box-like, good-gas-mileage minivan rolled off the assembly line, an entire generation of pedal-to-the-metal males has been unceremoniously eased into the lane of life marked, "Slower Vehicles Keep Right."

But, if you have kids, especially more than one, chances are that you will someday be behind the wheel of a minivan, whose introduction wiped out entire facets of male behavior.

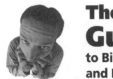
Chapter Eleven

Dodge Caravan owners do not shop for mag wheels or glasspack mufflers. No one speed-shifts the Ford Windstar through rush-hour traffic. Nobody in the gas pedal-tromping history of high-octane premium unleaded has ever shouted, "Eat my dust!" from the driver's seat of a Chrysler Town & Country.

Had James Dean rocketed off into eternity while behind the wheel of a minivan, even with the luggage rack and extra cup holders, his legacy of cool would have rivaled that of Barry Manilow.

That's not to say minivans are not without their advocates, such as single men who wish to remain that way. When it comes to keeping the opposite sex safely at a distance, minivans are in a class of their own. Nothing works quite like rolling down the standard-equipment power window and shouting, "Hi girls, it's Mr. Practical."

And, if nothing else, minivans are exactly that – practical.

When it comes to hauling the sheer tonnage of childhood, minivans are practical in spades.

When it comes to 47 weekly trips to the grocery store, minivans are the double-bagged, meat-and-potatoes of practical. When it comes to cross-country vacations, minivans are the take-everything-we-own, rolling-storage-shed of practical. When it comes to being parked in your own driveway, minivans are boring as all get out.

But, just when it appeared you had automatically shifted into terminal suburban bland, a quintet of Texas-based musical lunatics known as the Austin Lounge Lizards gave minivan males a complete testosterone overhaul.

Basically, the Austin Lounge Lizards are the epitome of eclectic, your basic bad boys of bluegrass who present music for the hard of thinking in intricate four- or five-part harmony.

Nothing is sacred in Lizard land where song titles include "Life is Hard, But Life Is Hardest When You're Dumb" and "Put The Oak Ridge Boys In The Slammer."

Cool Cars: A Thing Of The Past

Now, in the musical span of three minutes and forty four seconds, the Austin Lounge Lizards have once again made it acceptable, no make that downright enjoyable, to slide your suburban, stressed-out-father-of-two posterior behind the wheel.

From the opening strains, "Hey, Little Minivan" is classic pseudo-Beach Boys at their car song best, albeit with the Lounge Lizard's patented demented spin.

"On deadman's curve, I used to shut 'em down, I had the hottest muscle car in my hometown

I could burn rubber in all four gears, but I haven't done that in a million years

Hey, little minivan, we're goin' to the grocery store"

The first time I popped the Lizards' CD "Employee of the Month" in the player, I was in mid-mope, with our children in uncooperative tow for an afternoon of weekend errands. By the time, "Hey, Little Minivan," was through, they were questioning dad's sanity.

With each and every high-harmony chorus, I could feel my sing-along male batteries recharging. I hit the repeat button, then hit it again and then a third time.

By the fourth time through the song, I was driving like the proverbial maniac, zipping along at almost three, maybe even four miles over the posted speed limit. If I remember correctly, I think I even told the kids to, "hang on," as I brazenly switched lanes without using the blinker.

As we shot past a bewildered woman in her foreign sports car in the Pick 'n Save parking lot, I couldn't help it and gave the driver's side power window a shot.

"Hey, eat my dust!!!"

Boy, it was good to be back.

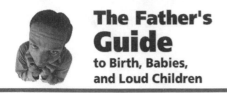
Chapter Eleven

The Automotive King
Of Double Dorkiness

Like many males, I secretly had hoped to complete the trifecta of male immaturity by somehow, someway, someday adding "Harley owner" to a resume that already included sportswriter and mid-life musician.

After the first minivan put those hopes on the ropes, the dreams of cruising atop a gleaming, chrome-covered Harley-Davidson were put down for the count by the addition of the second minivan.

In terms of automotive tedium, the only thing more boring than a minivan in your driveway is two minivans. Unless, of course, it happens to be not only two minivans, but two almost identical minivans, parked side-by-side as a symbol of full-blown suburban surrender in the battle of substance versus style.

Thanks to the natural demise of a we-got-our-money's-worth Toyota Camry that dated back to the administration of Father Bush, we found ourselves in need of immediate vehicular augmentation.

A line-by-line jaunt through the Sunday automotive section dangled the lure of a return to highway hipness, seducing the average male torque dork with cool-sounding car names such as Prowler, Cruiser and the pipedream of all pre-children pipedreams, the Corvette.

A line-by-line jaunt through the checkbook, bolstered by a glance at the toy-littered living room, immediately dismissed any thoughts of chrome-plated trendiness.

With three children under the age of 7 putting us three children beyond a two-seat convertible, we focused on simple criteria – interior stain resistance, number of cup holders, print size on the inevitable recall notice and, above all, the ability to haul stuff, stuff and more stuff.

The choice between another minivan and anything else with an engine and four tires was really no choice at all. While practicality narrowed our choices primarily to minivans, limited patience for auto shopping steered us down the road of familiarity.

Cool Cars: A Thing Of The Past

At the risk of sounding like a commercial (or possibly angling for a free minivan from the wonderful folks in the Chrysler Corp. marketing department who obviously realize the tremendous public relations value of this endorsement) we simply turned toward what had worked for us in the past.

The decision between purchasing a new minivan or a used minivan was based on simple economics. Unless one of the many storage places (or as our friends at Chrysler would like to hear, one of the many extremely useful, well-placed, easy-to-clean storage spaces) in the old minivan was unknowingly stuffed with freshly laundered 20 dollar bills, we would probably be pounding the pavement of the used car lot.

With much of the pre-shopping decision-making done, the actual shopping required about 17 minutes of intense scrutiny of a lot full of minivans.

We were down to the all-important coin flip to decide between forest green and white when the salesman mentioned an incoming minivan that had yet to be placed on the lot.

In terms of mileage and price, it seemed to be exactly what we were looking for. In terms of boring, it was the exact same boring color and boring style as the boring minivan currently occupying a boring space in our boring driveway.

Aside from being a year newer, the only noticeable difference was that the new van had a rooftop luggage rack, the one accessory that makes unhip even more unhip.

Inside, the new van had four adult chairs instead of the built-in kids' seats and some sort of rear air vents. Other than that, they were both candy apple red with a gray interior.

From the kids' standpoint, however, the distinction was not only evident, it was worth fighting for.

"OK, guys, get in the van."

"WE WANNA TAKE THE NEW VAN!!"

"But, it's the same as the old van."

"NO, IT'S NOT ... IT'S NEW!!"

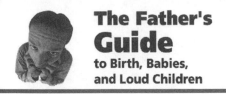
Chapter Eleven

"OK, guys, get in the new van."

"I GET TO SIT IN THE BACK ... YOU ALWAYS GET TO SIT IN THE BACK ... DO NOT ... DO TOO ... DO NOT ... DO TOO ..."

"OK, guys, get out of the van."

In addition to 57.3 times more room than the recently deceased Camry, another benefit of the boring similarity between the two vans is interchangeable parts, including the seats.

To put the new van through its paces, we opted for the time-honored weekend road trip, switching the kids' seats into the new van. Some 300 miles later, the interior of the new van looked remarkably like that of the old van, littered with candy wrappers, bread crumbs, bits of french fries, used Kleenex and all of the other mini-baggage generated by a family excursion.

With a summer of family outings looming on the horizon and a driveway full of interchangeable seats, we are ready for almost anything the road can throw our way.

As such, I am the mental savior for many fathers of young children whose minivan existence calls in to question their standing among their automotive peers. Thanks to our two minivans, no other dad on the highway can possibly be as dorky as I am.

Chapter Twelve

The More
The Merrier

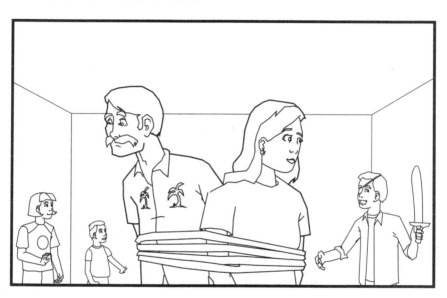

The Parental Refresher Course

Continuing education may be a necessity in the rung-by-rung climb up the corporate ladder, but when it comes to parenting, there is absolutely nothing refreshing about the refresher course.

Much had changed in the three years between our second and third kids. Colin arrived as an almost-10 pound memory-jogging package of hourly nursing, newborn diapers and sleepless nights when he checked in healthy, happy and hungry almost three years to the day after his older brother.

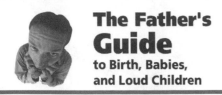

Chapter Twelve

We had not ruled out a third child, so in eventual preparation, we had at one time carefully boxed, labeled and packed away several tons of bottles, nipples, blankets, baby sacks, bassinet toys and mom and dad's anti-crabby pills. Over the maternity-free span of 36 months, however, we had managed to misplace, mislabel or misuse the entire warehouse of newborn necessities.

Boxes clearly labeled "baby clothes" in the blackest block lettering of the thickest, most permanent Magic Marker known to man had somehow switched contents with one of the Christmas ornament boxes. Colin might not be well-dressed, but he's at least well-decorated.

Over the same 36-month period, dozens of rebellious screws had one by one separated themselves from the pack of other screws during a variety of household projects. Somewhere in this house, one renegade screw literally holds the 3-year-old secret to re-assembling an infant swing.

Fortunately for us, Hayley, had become our household memory bank. She is the official designated finder in charge of cataloging and collecting on a daily basis all things lost over the previous 24 hours, including, but not limited to, car keys, half-full coffee cups and parental sanity.

Preparation for an additional child was not just limited to the mental aspects of parenting. Over the course of stumbling through life on auto pilot, my body, like that of many similarly aged males, had conveniently and contentedly fooled itself into thinking it is has remained in the exact same (i.e. nearly-Olympian) shape over that three-year span without the aid of a single sit-up.

Tom Carey, an outstanding songwriter from Illinois who has authored several books, best sums up this male phenomenon in his unabridged edition of *The Marriage Dictionary*.

His definition of "athlete" is: 'What your husband still sees when he looks in the mirror." This is followed by "athlete's foot," which is: "The only part of your husband that is still truly athletic."

Participation of friends and family also is an important part of the refresher curriculum.

As news spread of Colin's arrival, lifelong friends were quick to call. Voices similar in age to mine clearly stated, "Congratulations," but the

The More The Merrier

tone was unmistakably, "ARE YOU NUTS???" Most of them were laughing as they hung up.

Family members also jumped into the well-wishing spirit, consistently calling on the telephone exactly three minutes after Colin had gone to sleep. After fussing for another 40 minutes, Colin went back to sleep. Two minutes later, well-intentioned neighbor children would ring the front door bell, wishing to "see the baby."

Turning off the telephone ringers and taping over the doorbell with a sign that says, "Baby sleeping, come back in six months," is the first required assignment for any parental refresher course.

Thanks to Colin, we also refreshed ourselves on the usual array of newborn topics, including sleep deprivation and its effects; refereeing sibling rivalry; history of the seven-minute nap; stain removal – synthetics versus cotton; and the ever-popular arc diameter of the diaper-changed male.

But, after a short while, we obviously started to get the hang of it again. After all, we've made it this far.

Putting The Sibling In Rivalry

When it comes to newborn babies, first-time parents will have no clue. Second-time parents will have no chance.

First-born children are welcomed with open arms by wholly unprepared, but giddy, adults, whose previously structured lives will happily disintegrate into the daily trial-and-error method of on-the-job parental training.

It is blissful ignorance at its best, misery at its happiest.

Integrating a newborn into a house where toddlers already have staked their toy-littered claim, however, is like carrying a torch into the room where the explosives are stored.

While first-time parents are in for a rude awakening (actually many, many rude awakenings), they smilingly stumble and bumble from one sleepless night through one disaster-filled day after another. They will stagger around like zombies, but they are happy zombies. First-time parents are the Ward and June Cleaver of zombies.

"Hey!! We got two straight hours of sleep. Isn't it great? And those dark circles under your eyes go so well with that blouse."

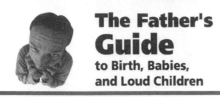

Chapter Twelve

Having a new baby for the first time means having no routine. No schedule is the schedule. Everybody is on the same page, although the pages are in random order.

Eventually, some sort of consistent calm will settle upon the household with just enough structure to conflict with everything else upon the arrival of the next child.

It is the quintessential showdown. "This town ain't big enough for both of us." There is a reason why the phrase sibling rivalry begins with sibling.

First-time parents are exhausted, but there actually are occasions where, when the baby naps, the parents nap. There is a recorded instance of this in Tennessee in 1968 and another one in France in 1989. This is never the case in a multi-child family.

According to the *Official Toddler Handbook* (pain-in-the-rear edition), the single, solitary job of an older brother or sister is to make enough noise to wake a sleeping baby. A truly dedicated toddler will be able to accomplish this feat at any time, night or day. If, by some miracle, the baby actually nods off in the middle of the night, it will automatically activate the nightmare nerve in most toddlers, triggering an avalanche of blood-curdling screams. This will not only wake your baby, it will wake babies for miles around. Scaring the absolute bejeezus out of comatose parents merely piles up bonus points.

To combat daytime naps, making up and singing loud, off-key kid songs is the weapon of choice for most toddlers. If all else fails, jumping from a high place will usually do the trick. If the loud thump doesn't get them, the vibration will.

Toy stickers that read, "For ages 3 to 6," are actually toddler-understood coded messages that mean, "loud enough to wake your baby brother or sister."

When it comes to toddlers and infants in the same household, Sybil did not have enough personalities to cover the undivided attention that is required. When babies need attention, toddlers want it. When toddlers want it, babies need it.

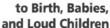

The More The Merrier

In the parental pecking order, need wins out over want. Patient toddlers file away this perceived slight and eventually extract their revenge in the form of out-of-style hand-me-downs.

New babies also bring out the helper in older siblings. This is the ultimate weapon for a toddler, whose help invariably creates more work for all concerned. A toddler-aided diaper change can last for hours with a clean-up normally associated with a chemical spill.

Requests of, "Can I hold the baby?" usually result in some sort of wrestling-style stranglehold. If two other siblings are involved, it immediately deteriorates into an arm-a-piece tug-of-war, culminating not only in everyone crying, but a couple of trips to the timeout chairs. Justice is swift in the court of sleep-deprived parents.

In addition to a couple of bedraggled adults, our house is populated by three children. The first two were 16 months apart with number three arriving almost exactly three years after the second one.

Friends who survive a visit to our house usually offer the polite commentary, "How do you do it?" What they really mean, as they scamper for safety of their cars, is "Why do you do it?" In our case, the answers speak for themselves, even if it is with a little bit of sassiness. And, or course, the answer is loud enough to wake a baby.

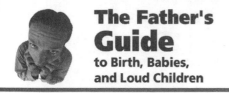

Chapter Twelve

Two's A Party, Three's A Stress Test

What we thought to be nothing more than simple addition turned out be an unsolvable parenting problem in long division.

After three years of adjusting to the you-take-one, I'll-take-the-other world of two children, Karen, and I figured the addition of a third child would be no more difficult than the simple flash-card arithmetic of two plus one equals three.

That is accurate if you're adding up the total number of future tuition payments. But if I correctly remember my pre-calculator old math (make that old, old, old math), the actual formula for determining the ratio of parent attention per child is two goes into three one time, subtract the one, carry the baby and the answer is 1 1/2 children per sleepless adult.

Mathematically correct, parentally impossible.

In real-life, the only time the phrase "half-child" applies is in reference to an adult male, usually in describing one of his hobbies. When it comes to parenting, however, the on-paper, long-division answer involving half a child may be technically correct, but in reality, the answer must be rounded up to the nearest toddler.

In other words, somebody is always outnumbered. The best parental odds you can get are 2-to-1. One parent is occupied with two children, while the other parent goes one-on-one with the remaining child, usually spent in a deep, meaningful, I'm-100-percent-serious lecture on not covering the dog with Play-Doh.

As a friend of mine and father of three recently pointed out, you have to switch from a man-to-man defense to a zone because you can't cover everybody.

The More The Merrier

For one thing, the youngest demands constant attention from one parent. In our case, the Colin day is divided equally between Karen and me. Karen is on Colin duty for 23 hours and 50 minutes, while I uncomplainingly step forward to assume the remaining 10 minutes, usually after being subtly reminded, "Could you hold him while I do (fill in the appropriate whatever)."

"Yes, dear (and according to my watch you now have nine minutes and 47 seconds remaining)."

When he was about three months old, Colin apparently subconsciously feared he would be stranded on a desert without liquids. As such, he nursed about 112 times a day, as he was obviously too small to carry a canteen.

Each nursing episode sent a clear pre-school signal to the other two kids that mom was occupied, now is the chance to misbehave.

Hayley and Tyler read the signal loud and clear. They knew that for the duration of the nursing session, they would have uninterrupted opportunity to spill, spray, splatter, splash and still think up an excuse as to how it all happened.

As all parents with three children know, there are two standard answers.

Hayley: "Tyler did it."

Tyler: "Hayley did it."

They didn't need to go to West Point to learn the divide-and-conquer strategy. Little do they know that the meter was running and the hours at which they will eventually be babysitting their younger brother for free are now being calculated per misdeed.

Compounding the jump from two children to three children is that the entire world is geared toward pairs, or at the very least, even-numbered everything.

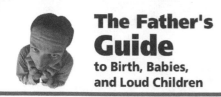
Chapter Twelve

Pull-along bike carts hold two children. Carnival rides seat two, side-by-side. One teeters, the other totters. Mounds bars have two mounds. Nobody ever offers a 3-for-the-price-of-2 coupon. Even in the crosswalk, there are only two adult hands to hold.

Another friend of mine, laughing with us not at us after Colin's arrival, said we will never, ever again be seated at a restaurant table in less than an hour. He has apparently made a lifelong study of watching countless "table for fours" be seated well ahead of the lone "table for five," regardless of which group arrived first.

I'm sure there must be government grant money available to further study the subject of "Third Children: The Cause Of Suburban Restaurant Hunger."

Actually, from what we heard from other parents of three is that our adjustment was fairly normal. Even Hayley and Tyler have gotten into the spirit of things, eagerly awaiting the day when they can capitalize on having a younger brother with the simple phrase: "COLIN DID IT!!"